Improving Speech Intelligibility in Adults

Clinical Application of Evidence-Based Strategies

Improving Speech Intelligibility in Adults

Clinical Application of Evidence-Based Strategies

Connie K. Porcaro, PhD, CCC-SLP

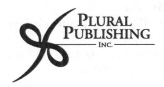

PLURAL
PUBLISHING
INC.

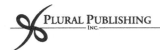

5521 Ruffin Road
San Diego, CA 92123

e-mail: information@pluralpublishing.com
Web site: https://www.pluralpublishing.com

Typeset in 11/13 ITC Garamond Std by Achorn International
Printed in the United States of America by McNaughton & Gunn, Inc.

Library of Congress Cataloging-in-Publication Data:

Names: Porcaro, Connie K., 1964- author.
Title: Improving speech intelligibility in adults : clinical application of
  evidence-based strategies / Connie K. Porcaro.
Description: San Diego, CA : Plural Publishing, Inc., 2022. | Includes
  bibliographical references and index.
Identifiers: LCCN 2022020932 (print) | LCCN 2022020933 (ebook) |
  ISBN 9781635503579 (paperback) | ISBN 1635503574 (paperback) |
  ISBN 9781635503586 (ebook)
Subjects: MESH: Speech Intelligibility | Speech Disorders--therapy |
  Evidence-Based Practice | Adult
Classification: LCC RC428.8 (print) | LCC RC428.8 (ebook) | NLM WV 501 |
  DDC 616.85/506--dc23/eng/20220728
LC record available at https://lccn.loc.gov/2022020932
LC ebook record available at https://lccn.loc.gov/2022020933

Contents

Preface

The most important gift we give our clients is the ability to be understood, to have their thoughts and requests heard. I've had the idea for this book in my heart and my head for many years. My interest in intelligibility began with a client who had a diagnosis of Amyotrophic Lateral Sclerosis (ALS). He was a big, tough biker with a large beard that covered much of his face. While he looked intimidating, he was a gentle giant. In dealing with his disease, he was frustrated by people not understanding him. I noticed I found him easier to understand on the phone than in person. This was near the time I began my doctoral studies, so I began questioning whether visual information was helpful when it comes to intelligibility in our clients.

When I started my doctoral program at the University of Arizona, I enrolled in courses and research experiences to learn as much as possible about speech perception and intelligibility. One semester, I worked in a psychology lab, running participants through a study of the McGurk effect, where the visual and auditory stimuli do not match. Listeners often have a different perception than what they are hearing based on the visual information. The McGurk effect is so strong that even if you are aware of it and know the stimuli don't match, it still influences your perception. I found this fascinating but had struggled to understand how it applies to our work with clients. But it brought me back to the client who I understood better when I wasn't looking at his face. I selected this topic for my dissertation research.

Once I dived into the literature on this topic, I was overwhelmed by the amount of research in the fields of speech-language pathology and audiology devoted to speech intelligibility. There are so many studies with different populations, including non-disordered speakers, speakers with hearing impairment, and speakers with dysarthria. It was difficult to make connections between studies because so many different measures and methods were employed. I completed my dissertation, which examined contributions of visual information to speech intelligibility in individuals with Parkinson's disease. It was a solid start to the rest of my career, in which my research and clinical work focused on improved intelligibility.

Soon after I presented my dissertation research at the Annual Convention of the American Speech-Language-Hearing Association in 2005, I was asked to present a session on intelligibility at the South Carolina Speech-Language-Hearing Association Convention. I decided the best way to present information on intelligibility to clinicians was to tie the research we have to what they are actively doing with clients. I used the studies on intelligibility and tied each section of my presentation to how clinicians could use the evidence from research to connect with best practices for their clients. This session was well-received, and I have presented it for many other state SLP associations as well. I found it very gratifying to speak with clinicians from all over the country about their adult clients with reduced intelligibility. I will never forget an SLP who approached me after my presentation in Ohio and told me he was glad I had given him strategies to use other than non-speech oral motor exercises. He told me he didn't really know there was anything else besides those exercises to help with intelligibility. That surprised me, but I realized that if SLPs don't know about the research on intelligibility, they may feel like they have few options for treating clients with reduced intelligibility. My goal with this book is to help bridge the gap between factors that influence intelligibility that we've learned from research and what works best clinically. I hope this book will provide clinicians with many suggestions and solutions, and induce more questions and thoughts on the topic.

This book allows for use of evidence-based practice by joining what we've learned from research to clinical judgment of SLPs and what works best for individual clients. There are literally thousands of research studies on intelligibility. I will not refer to them all, but I have shared topics you can use daily with your clients. I think it is common for SLPs to tie use of strategies and behavioral changes to clients when assessing and treating reduced intelligibility. While this book covers speaker factors thoroughly, my goal is to expand SLPs' thinking into other areas. Listeners or communication partners can also change behaviors and use strategies to ensure the message gets through. Even the environment where the communication takes place impacts intelligibility. We know about speaker, listener, and environmental factors from research, but don't always apply them to working with clients. Many of our clients may not be able to change their speech, but communicative partners can take some of the work involved to improve communication. And both partners can make changes to the environment to facilitate better exchange of information.

Chapter 1 introduces the components of intelligibility, including the triad of speaker, listener, and communication environment. Related concepts, including comprehensibility, efficiency, and speech naturalness are defined. Discussion of evidence-based practice in assessment and management sets the foundation to tie research into clinical work as explored in the other chapters.

In Chapter 2, the idea that both voice and speech disorders can reduce intelligibility is introduced. Disorders, signs, and symptoms related specifically to the speaker or client are described, along with the impact on reduced intelligibility. A subsystems approach is used to organize the information.

Chapter 3 considers the use of evidence-based practice to assess the structures and functions of our clients. Practical measurements of respiration, phonation, articulation, resonation, and prosody are described. Optimal recording methods are presented, including the best ways to record remotely for SLPs using telepractice with their clients.

The focus of Chapter 4 is on common-sense ways to most effectively and accurately measure intelligibility in adult clients. This chapter will provide SLPs with a clear idea of how to consider factors that can influence intelligibility measures they may use with clients. A checklist to remind SLPs of factors to consider when assessing intelligibility is included.

Management of the speaker's disorder through a subsystem approach is covered in Chapter 5. Supporting evidence is tied to strategies and tasks to improve intelligibility by altering the client's behavior.

Chapter 6 focuses on management based on strategies specifically found to improve intelligibility and comprehensibility. Practical suggestions and a checklist for speakers are provided.

Chapter 7 describes strategies that listeners can use to better understand speakers with reduced intelligibility. There is an emphasis on the speaker and listener working together. A checklist is provided for listeners along with suggestions for SLPs to work with both communicative partners, based on research findings.

Chapter 8 contains basic ideas about how the communication environment affects the ability of a listener to understand a speaker's message. Strategies for solving challenges related to the communication environment that can be detrimental to intelligibility are presented. Information related to use of face masks is discussed and a checklist is included to remind both communication partners to modify the environment for optimal communication.

Being understood is everything to our clients.

Acknowledgments

Much of the credit for my research interest and the idea for this book lies with clients I have worked with over the years. I would like to acknowledge former and current colleagues who reinforced my efforts on this book and contributed to my knowledge about the wide topic of intelligibility. Several individuals supported me enormously and my deepest thanks goes to the following people:

Dr. Kate Bunton for originally sustaining my dissertation research during good and challenging times, as well as for her review and helpful comments on chapters of this book.

Dr. Paul Evitts for providing resources related to Head and Neck Cancer and general support of my research and this book.

Dr. Katie Hustad for contributing tremendously to research in intelligibility. Also, for providing excellent suggestions and edits on assessment topics and chapter review of this book.

Dr. Paul Blanchett for reviewing chapters, offering suggestions, and reviewing the cases in each chapter. His assistance was quick, thoughtful, and always supportive.

Melanie Leisen for editing carefully and demonstrating phenomenal skills with APA while working as my graduate assistant. Her assistance was truly time-saving and invaluable to me.

Dr. Teresa Ukrainetz for mentoring me through my PhD and all of my jobs and projects since then. Her support and encouragement kept me going.

I am thankful for and grateful to the editorial team at Plural Publishing, who supported my idea for this book and for their editing assistance

XX   IMPROVING SPEECH INTELLIGIBILITY IN ADULTS

through the process. Many thanks to Valerie Johns, Christina Gunning, and Emily Pooley for all their help.

The many hours researching and writing this book cut into my family's togetherness at times, but they have been patient and encouraging. I am fortunate to have two close family members, my son Alex and daughter-in-law Alexa, who are SLPs. I appreciate that I can discuss topics related to the field with them. And, I gratefully acknowledge that my son Cameron and husband Mike don't always want to hear these SLP conversations but are always positive and supportive of my writing endeavors.

This work is dedicated to the many researchers who have studied intelligibility over the years and to the clinicians who can change clients' lives using this knowledge.

CHAPTER 1

Introduction of Intelligibility and Related Concepts

Key Points:

- When we add contextual information or cues (comprehensibility) to what a speaker says (intelligibility), listeners understand more.

- Improving a client's naturalness or efficiency of speech may reduce intelligibility, so it's important to determine priorities with our clients to consider these trade-offs.

- Intelligibility is impacted by the speaker, listener, and communication environment, as well as shared experiences, context, and knowledge.

- Assessment and management of clients with reduced intelligibility should focus on the physical cause of the disorder, activity limitations, and restriction on their ability to participate in typical daily life.

- Implementation science and evidence-based practice can assist SLPs in using research findings to improve our clients' ability to communicate.

Think for a moment about the one goal that applies to most, if not all, the clients you've worked with as a speech-language pathologist (SLP). The answer likely includes improving the client's ability to communicate their ideas, wants, and needs. The primary goal for our clients is to have listeners understand them. In cases related to speech or voice, this often involves the concept of intelligibility. When SLPs discuss intelligibility, we are describing a listener's understanding of the speaker's message (Duffy, 2019). We may associate intelligibility with young children with speech sound disorders or possibly older clients with dysarthria. However, clients with reduced intelligibility will have different etiologies, disorders, and ages. Speech disorders often cause reduced intelligibility, but voice disorders can also reduce what listeners understand (Evitts et al., 2016; Porcaro et al., 2020). Whereas challenges related to the speaker can reduce intelligibility, SLPs should consider factors related to listeners and the environment that can also impact whether a message is communicated (Yorkston et al., 1996). Using careful assessment to determine what is contributing to our clients' functional impairment is especially important in cases of reduced intelligibility. This book ties current research knowledge to assessment and management of reduced intelligibility in adult clients. It includes general concepts to target increased intelligibility, regardless of etiology or disorder, and focuses on all aspects related to an exchange of information between communication partners.

DEFINITIONS OF INTELLIGIBILITY, COMPREHENSIBILITY, AND RELATED MEASURES

Intelligibility

We commonly define intelligibility as the degree to which the speaker's intended message is recovered by the listener (Kent et al., 1989). This definition concerns the acoustic signal, or what we could capture using a recording device. The speaker's ability to correctly produce speech sounds can affect this auditory signal. In this way, the speaker's movements and coordination will affect the acoustic signal. Speakers with impaired speech may use strategies to alter the signal. These strategies may be innate behaviors that the client has started using or may be something that he or she learned previously in speech therapy. For example, if a client tried using a slower rate and feedback from listeners indicated they understood at the slower rate, then that may be a strategy they use routinely. In assessment and management of intelligibility, it is critical to consider how strategies can improve what the listener understands.

Comprehensibility

Comprehensibility is the degree to which a listener understands the speaker's message, based not only on the acoustic signal, but also using other available information. Yorkston and colleagues (1996) describe comprehensibility as a type of intelligibility that involves consideration of context. Comprehensibility, also known as contextual intelligibility, involves the consideration of both signal-dependent and signal-independent information. Signal-dependent information is the acoustic signal that leaves the speaker's mouth and travels to the listener's ears. The acoustic signal is what we define as intelligibility, and this is illustrated in Figure 1–1. Factors related to the speaker include their specific impairment, but also include any compensatory strategies that person may use. The combination of these is processed by the listener and the outcome is intelligibility.

Comprehensibility adds signal-independent information to what the listener uses in understanding the message (Yorkston et al., 1996). Comprehensibility, shown in Figure 1–2, includes the factors related to the acoustic signal and intelligibility, but also adds signal-independent factors. Signal-independent information includes shared knowledge of the topic or context cues. A listener will have an advantage if they know the topic of conversation is today's weather, as they will be able to listen for weather-related words even if the speaker's acoustic signal is difficult to understand. The same speaker could add a gesture showing "rain" or "umbrella" to help the listener follow their message. Use of these signal-independent strategies represents real-life communication where speakers and listeners can enhance understanding to improve comprehensibility.

As one might expect, the additional information provided by comprehensibility may lead to greater listener understanding compared to intelligibility (Hustad, 2008). However, these two measures, which seem very similar, have not been found to be independently related. Fontan and colleagues (2015) investigated the relationship between intelligibility and comprehension in background noise and reported that in functional communication situations, intelligibility scores did not predict listener comprehension. These findings show that we should not assume a person's intelligibility score will indicate how well listeners will comprehend what they say. One common factor that seems to be related to both intelligibility and comprehensibility is the severity of the individual's speech disorder. In fact, no significant relationship has been found between intelligibility and comprehensibility when the third variable of severity is controlled (Hustad, 2008). The relationship among these variables indicates that as severity increases, intelligibility and comprehensibility both decrease (Weismer & Martin, 1992). Because comprehensibility is a type of intelligibility that involves context, for the purposes of this book, "intelligibility" will mainly be a general term that will include comprehensibility. There

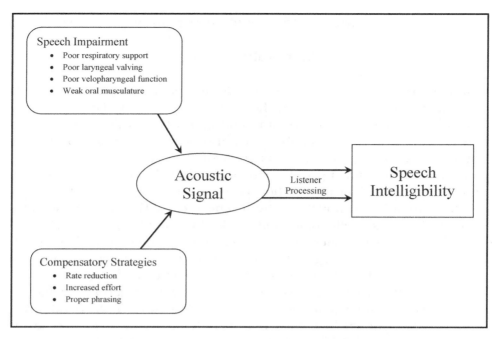

Figure 1–1. A model of factors that contribute to the adequacy of the acoustic signal and, therefore, to the speech intelligibility of dysarthric individuals. Reproduced with permission from *American Journal of Speech-Language Pathology* 5(1), (1996). Copyright 1996, American Speech-Language-Hearing Association.

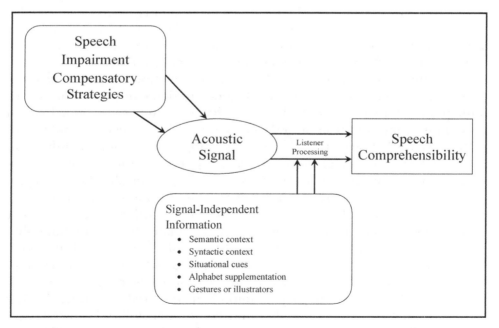

Figure 1–2. A model of factors that contribute to comprehensibility of dysarthric individuals. Reproduced with permission from *American Journal of Speech-Language Pathology* 5(1), (1996). Copyright 1996, American Speech-Language-Hearing Association.

will be specific examples, in chapters related to assessment and management, where the terms will be considered individually.

Efficiency

Efficiency is used to describe the rate at which the listener can understand information provided by the speaker (Duffy, 2019). This is an important measure to consider when evaluating either intelligibility or comprehensibility. In order to functionally manage reduced intelligibility, we need to know if the speaker's rate distracts or is noticeably slow to listeners. Some speakers may be intelligible to others only when using an unnaturally slow rate of speech. If the person can get the message across but not in a socially acceptable amount of time, then there is a negative impact on efficiency. A listener's comprehension may increase if a speaker uses an alphabet board to point to the first letter of each word they produce (Hustad & Lee, 2008). Although this may increase comprehensibility, the efficiency is decreased because this process will take longer. The balance of these factors is an important consideration in management.

Duffy (2019) describes the concepts of intelligibility, comprehensibility, and efficiency (ICE) and suggests that we consider all three as factors during assessment and management in speakers with dysarthria. Duffy's application of ICE was intended for individuals with motor speech disorders. However, these concepts are also useful with other disorder areas encountered in adult clients resulting in reduced intelligibility, including those with voice disorders.

Naturalness

Speech is natural "if it conforms to the listener's standards of rate, rhythm, intonation, stress patterning, and if it conforms to the syntactic structure of the utterance being produced" (Yorkston et al., 2010, p. 288). Duffy (2019) describes the use of stress and prosody as helpful in improving intelligibility. It is important to consider both naturalness and intelligibility when we work with clients as these concepts can be related. A person can be highly intelligible but their speech may call attention to them because it sounds "odd." For example, take the sentence, "The parrot is in the tree." If spoken with excessive pauses in between each word, the listener may become distracted by the unnatural pauses and miss the intended message. Research also demonstrates that speakers with dysarthria who have reduced intelligibility also receive poorer ratings of speech naturalness (Yorkston et al., 1990). The goal of treatment may be to increase intelligibility, but some strategies, such as slowing the rate of speech, may have a positive impact on intelligibility, but a negative impact on naturalness

(Rosenbek, 1984). Although our goal may be to increase intelligibility, the impact of the relationship between intelligibility and naturalness is an important clinical consideration.

Communicative Participation

Most of our daily activities, including work, family, education, and social activities, involve communicating with others. Communicative participation is defined as "taking part in life situations where knowledge, information, ideas or feelings are exchanged" (Eadie et al., 2006, p. 309). This definition includes all forms of communication, speaking, writing, listening, or reading, as well as nonverbal communication. Yorkston and Baylor (2011) point out that the word "exchange" in this definition indicates the responsibility speakers and listeners share to ensure that effective communication takes place. Determining a client's communicative participation can allow SLPs to facilitate the most functional, client-specific change to improve communication.

COMPONENTS OF A COMMUNICATION EXCHANGE

Examining the components of a communication exchange allows us to consider all of the factors that might impact intelligibility. These components are introduced in this chapter and discussed in more detail in later chapters of this book. We may think about intelligibility as "belonging" to the speaker, but there can be listener and environmental factors involved as well. In order to functionally assess and manage intelligibility, SLPs should consider all factors.

Theories of Communication

There are several theories of communication that provide terms to describe this process. At the most basic level of communication, one person shares a vocal message with another person. Although that definition is a good start, we can learn from communication models to add components that represent a more complete communication exchange. This enables us to more thoroughly examine all aspects of information exchange between our clients and their communication partners to provide effective management. Shannon and Weaver (1949) originally proposed the linear model of communication, which describes a sender (speaker) transmitting a message through a channel to a receiver (listener). This model also considered the concept of noise or factors that could interfere with the exchange of information. The interactional model of communication added feedback from the listener to the speaker (Schramm, 1954). The addition of feedback means

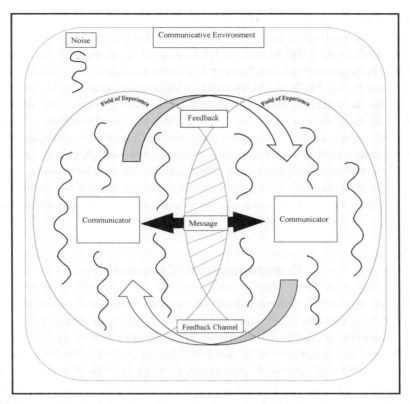

Figure 1–3. Factors related to effective communication featured in the transactional model of communication (Barnlund, 2008).

that both speakers and listeners are responsible for the effectiveness of the communication exchange. This model also considered that the speaker and listener would have different fields of experience, related to their own context, and understanding of the world. The transactional model did not describe speakers and listeners, but instead explained that both are best described as communicators because their roles would be switching rapidly during a conversation (Barnlund, 2008). The transactional model focuses on the need for shared overlap in the field of experiences of the communicators for effective communication, as illustrated in Figure 1–3. Messages are considered to be interdependent because what one person communicates may alter how the other person responds. The transactional model considers the interference of noise related to speaker, listener, and environment.

Feedback

When feedback is part of the exchange, the communicators move back and forth in the roles of speaker and listener. A second message responding to the first is an example of verbal feedback. So, if someone asks, "How are you?" and you respond, "I am well," your communication partner is certain that you understood the message. Inclusion of feedback in the model is a much better representation of everyday communication situations. People provide feedback both verbally and nonverbally. Feedback can provide reinforcement, such as when the listener nods to show the speaker he or she understood or agrees. In other cases, the feedback may serve as a request for more information. A response of "Huh?" is a verbal message to the speaker that the listener did not understand. A puzzled look can be a nonverbal way of expressing that we do not understand a message. Feedback is a critical part of a communication exchange because it allows the speaker to know if the message was understood and prompts the next response.

Communication Channels

People use different channels to send messages. Some channels are one-way, such as radio or television that involve no interaction between the speaker and the listener. In comparison, during two-way communication, we exchange information back and forth using verbal or written messages or gestures. We can transmit messages face-to-face or through a device, such as a computer or a cell phone. We utilize electronic channels, such as messages sent by e-mail or text. People also communicate messages through nonverbal channels, such as body language or facial expressions which can, at times, be as important in the message as the actual words (Giles & Le Poire, 2006). There may be situations where communication allows people to hear a speaker's message at a future time, using recorded speech. As the topic of this book is speech intelligibility, there is a focus on verbal messages, although examples for backup channels, such as writing or gestures which can aid communication, are addressed.

Communication Noise

Noise refers to anything that interferes with the message sent between the participants in a communication exchange. Noise can originate from the speaker, the communication environment, or even from the listener. There are four kinds of noise to consider during a communication exchange: physical, physiological, psychological, and semantic (Rothwell, 2016).

Physical Noise

Physical noise is a stimulus external to either communication partner that can prevent effective transmission of a message. This noise could distract the speaker from formulating the message clearly. It could impact the listener by interfering with the ability to hear the auditory signal from the speaker. There are many examples, including background noise from people talking or from a noisy fan. Physical noise could also involve distractions, such as poor lighting that does not allow the listener to see the speaker's face. Wearing masks reduces our ability to make the best use of both auditory and visual information from speakers (Kim & Thompson, 2021).

Physiological Noise

Physiological noise occurs when a message doesn't get communicated correctly because of a physiological issue within either the speaker or listener. The most obvious examples might be dysarthria, impairing the speaker's ability to articulate clearly, or a listener who cannot receive a message due to a hearing impairment. But other types of physiological noise could also prove to be a distraction and thus, influence a communication exchange. For example, either communication partner may feel ill or exhausted so they have difficulty producing or attending to the message. It is not always possible to eliminate the noise related to physiological noise, but it is necessary to be aware of its presence in a communication situation.

Psychological Noise

Psychological noise involves a mental interference that can influence what the speaker or listener perceives. The listener may go into the communication exchange with a bias or assumption about a speaker, which affects how the message is interpreted. Perhaps an unfamiliar listener hears a speaker with dysarthria and makes negative assumptions about the person's abilities based on their speech. This may cause the listener to interpret and react differently, impacting the message sharing. Psychological noise may also occur when one or both communication partners get distracted mentally by another agenda. Someone might think ahead in the conversation about how they will answer so they don't really listen to their partner's response. Or we may be mentally making a shopping list in our head and this lack of attention may cause us to miss someone's message.

Semantic Noise

Semantic noise is a type of internal noise often caused by the sender of a message. Semantic noise can affect communication because the sender is using a code that is unfamiliar to the listener. An obvious example would be two people trying to communicate when they do not have a shared language. But even with shared language, semantic noise can be present. Someone might ask you to "Spill the tea" and if you know that slang term, you know they are actually asking you to share gossip. If you don't, the speaker's request may get lost. As SLPs, we take care to not use professional jargon with our clients. If we were to use technical jargon, our clients would likely not understand our meaning. However, we do feel comfortable using professional jargon with other SLPs so semantic noise is influenced by shared experience and knowledge.

Shared Experience Between Communicators

A final component of the interactive model of communication involves the field of experience of both listener and speaker. This refers to the shared knowledge, context, and experience that will help to provide meaningful interaction when there is an overlap between speaker and listener (Corey, 2009). Examples might include cultural background, geographic location, or personal experiences (Rothwell, 2016). Both the speaker and listener will come to the conversation with their own field of experience. In most cases, there will be some overlap between the two, which will improve their ability to communicate. We can use this overlap to communicate more effectively, especially when the speaker is difficult to understand. The overlap of the speaker's and the listener's fields of knowledge, outlined with diagonal lines in Figure 1–3, shows us a shared field of experience. Different speaker-listener combinations will have various overlapping shared knowledge. SLPs know how valuable this shared knowledge can be in a communication exchange.

IMPAIRED COMMUNICATION

A breakdown in intelligibility can occur within any of the components related to the exchange of communication. Obviously, as SLPs, we are most familiar with a speaker with impairment. Our clients may experience reduced intelligibility as a result of various disorders, including dysarthria, apraxia, and even voice disorders. Here, the listener may be perfectly capable of understanding speech, and the communication environment may be suitable, but the message is flawed at the outset because of the speech/voice disorder. Sometimes, the communication environment is the problem. Perhaps a speaker without a disorder wants to send a message to a listener with adequate hearing abilities in a faulty communication environment, such as talking on a cell phone with poor reception ("Can you hear me now?"). This can result in a message that does not reach the listener as intended. Finally, the listener might be the source of the breakdown in communication. This situation may occur when a typical speaker provides an intact message through an effective environment, but the listener cannot receive the signal, perhaps due to a hearing impairment. Any of the types of noise mentioned earlier can also reduce the effectiveness of a communication exchange. Lack of shared experience or knowledge may contribute to a reduced understanding of a speaker's message. It is important to remember that any combination of these breakdowns can occur and all areas should be considered as we work with clients and their communication partners.

CONSIDERATION OF FUNCTION AND DISABILITY RELATED TO INTELLIGIBILITY

Reduced intelligibility can negatively affect the ability to participate in communication effectively for social, educational, and vocational purposes (Lowit & Kent, 2011). In order to consider function and disability related to intelligibility, we can apply the World Health Organization (WHO) framework, called the International Classification of Functioning, Disability and Health or ICF (World Health Organization, 2001). The ICF framework provides an interdisciplinary set of terms to describe the impact of health conditions, such as those that impair intelligibility. Table 1–1 illustrates the components of the ICF and provides examples related to intelligibility.

To illustrate the framework, I will briefly explain the four major components. A case study will be described in future chapters that connect a client with reduced intelligibility to these four components. The first component is impairment, referring to difficulties with the structures or the functions of the structures involved in speech production. For instance, in a patient with amyotrophic lateral sclerosis (ALS), the velum and articulators may not have normal movements. The second component is activity limitation, which refers to difficulty completing a task, in this case producing intelligible speech. Reduced intelligibility resulting from hypernasality and articulatory deficits may limit this person's activity. The third component is participation restriction, which refers to difficulty taking part in life situations. A person with ALS may have difficulty continuing to work and may not be able to participate in other activities requiring communication. It is important to remember that the amount of restriction will differ from client to client, even though their levels of impairment may look quite similar. Some people are more affected than others when reduced intelligibility or comprehensibility diminishes their ability to participate fully in their typical lives. The last component in the ICF, environmental factors, considers the communication environment in which the client is speaking. These factors can include such things as background noise and any issues related to the communication partner's ability to retrieve the spoken message. Appendix 1–1 provides a list of references for application of ICF to specific disorders where reduced intelligibility is expected.

Table 1–1. Consideration of ICF Framework in Intelligibility

ICF Components	Definition	Examples Related to Intelligibility
Body functions	Physiological and psychological functions of body systems	Speech systems, including respiration, phonation, articulation, and resonation
Body structures	Anatomical parts of the body	Respiratory system: lungs, trachea Phonatory system: larynx, vocal folds Articulatory system: lips, tongue, jaw Resonatory system: velum, upper airways
Impairments	Problems in body function and/or structure	Respiratory system: limited air for phonation Phonatory system: incoordination of vocal fold vibrations Articulatory system: slow, imprecise movements of tongue Resonatory system: lack of adequate closure of the velopharyngeal port
Activity	Execution of a task or action	Speaking
Participation	Involvement in a life situation	Speaking as needed for all life situations, including work, social, family obligations
Activity limitations	Difficulties in executing activities	Difficulty speaking so that others understand the speaker's wants, needs, and intentions = reduced intelligibility and/or comprehensibility
Participation restrictions	Problems participating in life situations	Difficulty speaking in situations specific to the person's life
Environmental factors	Physical, social, and attitudinal aspects of one's life *(may be barriers or facilitators)	Environmental factors, background noise, listener challenges or strategies

Note: Data compiled from Dykstra et al. (2007) and World Health Organization (2001).

INTEGRATING SCIENCE AND CLINICAL PRACTICE TO IMPROVE INTELLIGIBILITY

As an SLP, when you think of a measure of intelligibility, what comes to mind? For many of us, it is an intelligibility statement that appears often in reports, "Justin was judged to be approximately 80% intelligible." This is a common way that SLPs have described intelligibility for years, as though intelligibility is something we can estimate. There are many factors that can change intelligibility for any given client. And the ability to change or alter intelligibility becomes a double-edged sword. The positive side is that we can change it, which is desirable for our clients' ability to improve communication effectiveness. On the negative side, we must control the many factors that can influence intelligibility during assessment. It would not be smart to measure intelligibility in a client at baseline using one method and then complete the follow-up measure using a different method. If we are not measuring intelligibility in a standard way, then any increase or decrease we find may be related to altered methods of measurement rather than true client changes. These are also important issues when we plan management for clients with reduced intelligibility.

Using Evidence-Based Practice for Clinical Decisions

There are many factors that can affect intelligibility that SLPs have learned about through research. The aim of this book is to present these factors clearly, related to carefully controlled research findings. The American Speech-Language-Hearing Association (ASHA) has endorsed the use of Evidence-Based Practice (EBP) in the clinical decision-making process (American Speech-Language-Hearing Association, 2005). This involves considering current research findings, in addition to clinical perspective based on experience and client preferences when determining the best management approaches. With the emphasis placed on research, it may be tempting to equate EBP with research findings alone. Current, reliable, well-constructed research studies add considerably to having the right knowledge to select the best options for clients, but it is only one component of EBP. Using your own clinical experience and intuition based on what strategies have proved successful with other clients is critical. Considering input from the client should serve as a driving force in clinical decision-making. Yorkston and Baylor (2019) describe how patients themselves are the best sources of input based on reports of their own communicative environment, signs and symptoms, and personal preferences regarding their communication disorder. These authors present a strong case for patient-centered data collection to determine the appropriateness of management programs.

In order to thoroughly consider all critical aspects in making the best management decisions, Tonelli (2001) suggests including two other factors. The first is physiologic rationale, which includes application of principles related to current understanding of bodily processes. Etiology is an important consideration here and SLPs should also give thought to the pathophysiology or disordered processes that result from a client's disease or injury. Some clients with reduced intelligibility have experienced a traumatic brain injury (TBI) or stroke. In some of these cases, improvement may occur spontaneously as the brain injury heals. Others may have a neurodegenerative disease, such as Parkinson's disease or ALS, where we expect a decline in motor skills, which may reduce intelligibility as the disease progresses. The second factor involves system features, such as cultural, economic, and legal facilitators or barriers. This might include issues like whether the client can afford to pay for the number of visits recommended or if he or she has transportation to a clinic. When we plan functional management for clients, we must consider these types of factors.

Steps involved in using EBP include: 1st determine your clinical question, 2nd find evidence regarding efficacy of treatment options, 3rd cautiously evaluate the source and relevancy of the findings you are reviewing, and 4th make your clinical decision on treatment based on the research, your clinical judgment, and relevant client factors (American Speech-Language-Hearing Association, n.d.a). The intent of this book is to present clinicians with factors related to all components of communication that can affect intelligibility. In chapters related to assessment and management, research findings can assist you in considering these aspects related to EBP. Researchers have investigated factors related to intelligibility and we have many answers about what impacts and, in some cases, improves intelligibility. The important goal of improving intelligibility does not have to be hit or miss or simple guesswork if we strategically consider factors related to the concept and the knowledge that we already possess in our field.

Exploring Our Role in Bridging Research to Clinical Practice

Most clinicians know that it can be challenging to implement what you read in a published article in a real-world clinical setting. Implementation science is an interdisciplinary field whose goal is to bridge the gap between research and clinical practice (Fixsen et al., 2005). Implementation science works to find factors that facilitate or hinder the use of research evidence in clinical practice and then manage those challenges so that clinicians can utilize EBP for the best outcome with clients (Fixsen et al., 2005). In order to make these connections, practicing clinicians can work together with researchers to ensure the methods explored in investigations are workable in real-world settings. For example, Feuerstein and colleagues (2018) completed a pilot study that paired practitioners working on early communication signals in young children with researchers using qualitative methodology. Their conclusions indicated strong value in researchers working together with practicing clinicians to understand challenges involved in practical settings. Douglas and Burshnic (2019) provide an excellent overview and strong incentives for SLPs to involve themselves in implementation science to facilitate better outcomes with clients.

Utilizing Technology Appropriately for Best Practice

Use of telepractice has increased dramatically in response to shortages of SLPs in rural settings and to restrictions during the pandemic. ASHA supports the use of telepractice and defines it as "the application of telecommunications technology to the delivery of speech language pathology and audiology professional services at a distance by linking clinician to client or clinician to clinician for assessment, intervention, and/or consultation" (ASHA, n.d.b). Use of telepractice can help SLPs and their clients overcome barriers to successful evaluation and management, including distance from treatment providers, difficulty for clients to travel to services, or shortages of providers (Cason & Cohn, 2014). A strong advantage gained in using telepractice is that clients can be seen in the functional environment and with the communication partners they encounter in their daily lives, which supports the WHO intervention framework (2001). We can also expand our ability to communicate with specific groups, such as a client and their physician at the same time.

Comparisons of face-to-face evaluation and management versus those services provided through telepractice have shown that there can be equal effectiveness in these service methods. Duffy and his colleagues at the Mayo Clinic (1997) conducted a study of various adult neurogenic disorders, including apraxia of speech, dysarthria, and dysphonia. These researchers concluded that in most cases, a functional assessment can be conducted at a distance. Over the years, our technology has improved and the research has expanded. In patients with Parkinson's disease and hyperkinetic dysarthria, assessments conducted face-to-face and online were comparable (Constantinescu et al., 2010). Studies of treatment of speech/voice in clients with Parkinson's disease have demonstrated the telepractice effectiveness of management as measured by increased vocal intensity (Covert et al., 2018; Griffin et al., 2018; Quinn et al., 2018; Theodoros et al., 2016).

Research on telepractice across different client populations has shown to be effective and, given the wide use of this practice currently, we can expect many more studies on this topic. Weidner and Lowman (2020) reviewed 31 studies examining SLPs' use of telepractice with adult clients and concluded that this is an appropriate service delivery model. These authors suggested further studies will provide useful information regarding the types of strategies and technologies that will result in best practice in our field. If you are considering telepractice, there are many published studies and resources available through ASHA. A useful publication by Grillo (2019) summarizes many areas related to reimbursement, ethical issues, and technology platforms suitable for telepractice in speech-language pathology. You can find current and frequently updated resources in ASHA's evidence map related to telepractice (ASHA, n.d.b). Although there may be quite a bit to navigate if you are considering starting to use telepractice, it could be a very useful tool to allow you to expand services to more clients in a functional manner.

SUMMARY

Taking information from many sources and working together as clinicians and researchers will allow us to assist people who have reduced intelligibility. This is a critical goal for many of our clients. Our society functions when people understand each other. Most education, work, and social situations involve being able to communicate verbally. Based on the definitions considered in this chapter, an SLP would set goals for clients to be intelligible, comprehensible, and effective natural-sounding communicators. When working toward these goals with clients, SLPs need to consider disability and function, which is different for each client we encounter. In clinical decision-making, we should include all aspects related to evidence-based practice, including current research findings, clinical judgment, and client preferences. Technology has improved our ability to provide effective, functional services for our clients. Our goal as SLPs is to help people functionally communicate in their environment, as needed. Knowing all factors that can affect assessment and management of intelligibility will allow clinicians to make the most informed choices for their clients' communication needs.

> Case Study Introduction: At the conclusion of each chapter, you will find two case studies illustrating how content from the chapter is used by SLPs working with clients who have reduced intelligibility, which restricts their participation and ability to function optimally in their everyday lives. The methods and procedures used by the SLPs are written to assist you in thinking about how to apply the information in the chapter to your clients. The two cases illustrate assessment and management of a dysarthria case, secondary to traumatic brain injury and a voice disorder related to age-related voice changes (presbyphonia).

REFERENCES

American Speech-Language-Hearing Association. (n.d.a). *Evidence-based practice*. https://www.asha.org/research/ebp/

American Speech-Language-Hearing Association. (n.d.b). Telepractice. *ASHA's Evidence Maps*. https://www2.asha.org/EvidenceMapLanding.aspx?id=858 9944872&recentarticles=false&year=undefined&tab=all

American Speech-Language-Hearing Association. (2005). *Evidence-based practice in communication disorders* [Position statement]. http://www.asha.org /policy

Barnlund, D. C. (2008). A transactional model of communication. In C. D. Mortensen (Ed.), *Communication theory* (2nd ed., pp. 47–57). Transaction Publishers. https://doi.org/10.4324/9781315080918

Cason, J., & Cohn, E. R. (2014). Telepractice: An overview and best practices. *Perspectives on Augmentative and Alternative Communication, 23*, 4–17. https://doi.org/10.1044/aac23.1.4

Constantinescu, G., Theodoros, D., Russell, T., Ward, E., Wilson, S. & Wootton, R. (2010). Assessing disordered speech and voice in Parkinson's disease: A telerehabilitation application. *International Journal of Language & Communication Disorders, 45* (6), 630–644. https:// DOI: 10.3109 /13682820903470569

Corey, A. M. (2009). Introducing communication. In T. Pierce (Ed.), *The evolution of human communication: From theory to practice* (pp. 1–39). Etre-Books Press.

Covert, L. T., Slevin, J. T., & Hatterman, J. (2018). The effect of telerehabilitation on missed appointment rates. *International Journal of Telerehabilitation, 10*(2), 65–72.

Douglas, N. F. & Burshnic, V. L. (2019). Implementation science: Tackling the research to practice gap in communication sciences and disorders. *Perspectives of the ASHA Special Interest Groups, 4*(1), 3–7. https://doi .org/10.1044/2018_PERS-ST-2018-0000

Duffy, J. R., Werven, G. W., & Aronson, A. E. (1997). Telemedicine and the diagnosis of speech and language disorders. *Mayo Clinic Proceedings, 72*(12), 1116–1122. https://doi.org/10.4065/72.12.1116

Duffy, J. R. (2019). *Motor speech disorders: Substrates, differential diagnosis, and management* (4th ed.). Elsevier Mosby.

Dykstra, A. D., Hakel, M. E., & Adams, S. G. (2007). Application of the ICF in reduced speech intelligibility in dysarthria. *Seminars in Speech and Language, 28*(4), 301–311. https://doi.org/10.1055/s-2007-986527

Eadie, T. L., Yorkston, K. M., Klasner, E. R., Dudgeon, B. J., Deitz, J. C., Baylor, C. R., . . . Amtmann, D. (2006). Measuring communication participation: A review of self-report instruments in speech-language pathology. *American Journal of Speech-Language Pathology, 15*(4), 307–320. https://doi.org /10.1044/1058-0360(2006/030)

Evitts, P. M., Starmer, H., Teets, K., Montgomery, C., Calhoun, L., Schulze, A. . . . Adams, L. (2016). The impact of dysphonic voices on healthy listeners: Listener reaction times, speech intelligibility, and listener comprehension. *American Journal of Speech-Language Pathology, 25*(4), 561–575. https://doi.org/10.1044/2016_AJSLP-14-0183

Feuerstein, J. L., Olswang, L. B., Greenslade, K. J., Dowden, P., Pinder, G. L. & Madden, J. (2018). Implementation research: Embracing practitioners' views. *Journal of Speech, Language, and Hearing Research, 61*(3), 645–657. https://doi.org/10.1044/2017_JSLHR-L-17-0154

Fixsen, D. L., Naoom, S. F., Blasé, K. A., Friedman, R. M., & Wallace, F. (2005). *Implementation research: A synthesis of the literature* [Monograph]. Tampa, FL: University of South Florida, Louis de la Parte Florida Mental Health Institute, The National Implementation Research Network. (FMHI Publication No. 231). https://nirn.fpg.unc.edu/resources /implementation-research-synthesis-literature

Fontan, L., Tardieu, J., Gaillard, P., Woisard, V., & Ruiz, R. (2015). Relationship between speech intelligibility and speech comprehension in babble noise. *Journal of Speech, Language, and Hearing Research, 58*(3), 977–986. https://doi.org/10.1044/2015_JSLHR-H-13-0335

Giles, H., & Le Poire, B. A. (2006). The ubiquity and social meaningfulness of nonverbal communication. In V. Manusov & M. L. Patterson (Eds.), *The SAGE handbook of nonverbal communication*. SAGE Publications. http://dx.doi.org/10.4135/9781412976152

Griffin, M., Bentley, J., Shanks, J., & Wood, C. (2018). The effectiveness of Lee Silverman Voice Treatment therapy issued interactively through an iPad device: A non-inferiority study. *Journal of Telemedicine and Telecare, 24*(3), 209–215.

Grillo, E.U. (2019). Building a successful voice telepractice program. *Perspectives of the ASHA Special Interest Groups, 4*(1), 100–110. https://doi .org/10.1044/2018_PERS-SIG3-2018-0014

Hustad, K. C. (2008). The relationship between listener comprehension and intelligibility scores for speakers with dysarthria. *Journal of Speech, Language, and Hearing Research, 51*(3), 562–573. https://doi.org/10.1044 /1092-4388(2008/040)

Hustad, K. C., & Lee, J. (2008). Changes in speech production associated with alphabet supplementation. *Journal of Speech, Language, and Hearing Research, 51*(6), 1438–1450. https://doi.org/10.1044/1092-4388(2008/07-0185)

Kent, R. D., Weismer, G., Kent, J. F., & Rosenbek, J. C. (1989). Toward phonetic intelligibility testing in dysarthria. *Journal of Speech and Hearing Disorders, 54*(4), 482–499. https://doi.org/10.1044/jshd.5404.482

Kim, Y., & Thompson, A. (2021, November 18–20). *Effects of face masks on speech acoustics and intelligibility* [Technical session]. Annual Convention of the American Speech-Language-Hearing Association, Washington D.C.

Lowit, A., & Kent, R. D. (2011). *Assessment of motor speech disorders*. Plural Publishing.

Porcaro, C. K., Evitts, P. M., King, N., Hood, C., Campbell, E., White, L., & Veraguas, J. (2020). Effect of dysphonia and cognitive-perceptual listener strategies on speech intelligibility. *Journal of Voice, 34*(5), 806.e7–806.e18. https://doi.org/10.1016/j.jvoice.2019.03.013

Quinn, R., Park, S., Theodoros, D., & Hill, A. J. (2018). Delivering group speech maintenance therapy via telerehabilitation to people with Parkinson's disease: A pilot study. *International Journal of Speech-Language Pathology, 21*(4), 385–394. https:// doi.org/10.1080/17549507.2018.1476918

Rosenbek, J. C. (1984). Treating the dysarthric talker. *Seminars in Speech and Language, 5*(4), 359–384. https://doi.org/10.1055/s-2008-1064294

Rothwell, J. D. (2016). *In the company of others: An introduction to communication*. (5th ed.). Oxford University Press.

Schramm, W. (1954). *The process and effects of mass communication*. University of Illinois Press.

Shannon, C. E., & Weaver, W. (1949). *The mathematical theory of communication*. University of Illinois Press.

Theodoros, D. G., Hill, A. J., & Russell, T. G. (2016). Clinical and quality of life outcomes of speech treatment for Parkinson's disease delivered to the home via telerehabilitation: A noninferiority randomized controlled trial. *American Journal of Speech-Language Pathology, 25*(2), 214–232. https:// doi.org/10.1044/2015_AJSLP-15-0005

Tonelli, M. R. (2001). The limits of evidence-based medicine. *Respiratory Care, 46*(12), 1435– 1440.

Weidner, K. & Lowman, J. (2020). Telepractice for adult speech-language pathology services: A systematic review. *Perspectives of the ASHA Special Interest Groups, 5*(1), 326–338. https://doi.org/10.1044/2019_persp-19-00146

Weismer, G., & Martin, R. E. (1992). Acoustic and perceptual approaches to the study of intelligibility. In R. D. Kent (Ed.), *Intelligibility in speech disorders: Theory, measurement, and management* (pp. 67–118). John Benjamins Publishing Company. https://doi.org/10.1075/sspcl.1.04wei

World Health Organization (2001). *International Classification of Functioning, Disability, and Health*. https://www.who.int/standards/classifications /international-classification-of-functioning-disability-and-health

Yorkston, K. M., & Baylor, C. R. (2011). Measurement of communicative participation. In R. D. Kent & A. Lowit (Eds.), *Assessment of motor speech disorders* (pp.123–139). Plural Publishing.

Yorkston, K. M., & Baylor, C. R. (2019). Patient-reported outcome measures: An introduction for clinicians. *Perspectives of the ASHA Special Interest Groups, 4*(1), 8–15. https://doi.org/10.1044/2018_PERS-ST-2018-0001

Yorkston, K. M., Beukelman, D. R., Strand, E. A., & Hakel, M. (2010). *Management of motor speech disorders in children and adults* (3rd ed.). Pro-Ed.

Yorkston, K. M., Hammen, V. L., Beukelman, D. R., & Traynor, C. D. (1990). The effect of rate control on the intelligibility and naturalness of dysarthric speech. *Journal of Speech and Hearing Disorders, 55*(3), 550–560. https:// doi.org/10.1044/jshd.5503.550

Yorkston, K. M., Strand, E. A., & Kennedy, M. R. (1996). Comprehensibility of dysarthric speech: Implications for assessment and treatment planning. *American Journal of Speech-Language Pathology, 5*(1), 55–66. https://doi .org/10.1044/1058-0360.0501.55

APPENDIX 1–1

References for ICF Application to Specific Disorders Related to Reduced Intelligibility

MOTOR SPEECH DISORDERS

Cunningham, B. J., Washington, K. N., Binns, A., Rolfe, K., Robertson, B. & Rosenbaum, P. (2017). Current methods of evaluating speech language outcomes for preschoolers with communication disorders: A scoping review using the ICF-CY. *Journal of Speech, Language, and Hearing Research, 60*(2), 447–464. https://pubs.asha.org/doi/10.1044/2016_JSLHR-L-15-0329

Dykstra, A. D., Hakel, M. E., Adams, S. G. (2007). Application of the ICF in reduced speech intelligibility in dysarthria. *Seminars in Speech and Language, 28*(4), 301–311. https://DOI: 10.1055/s-2007-986527

Larkins, B. (2007). The application of the ICF in cognitive-communication disorders following traumatic brain injury. *Seminars in Speech and Language, 28*(4), 334–342. https://DOI: 10.1055/s-2007-986530

McLeod S., & McCormack, J. (2007). Application of the ICF and ICF-children and youth in children with speech impairment. *Seminars in Speech and Language, 28*(4), 254–264. https://doi.org/10.1055/s-2007-986522

Murray, E. & Iuzzini-Seigel, J. (2017). Efficacious treatment of children with childhood apraxia of speech according to the International Classification of Functioning, Disability, and Health. *Perspectives of the ASHA Special Interest Groups, SIG 2, 2*(2), 61–76. https://doi.org/10.1044/persp2.SIG2.61

Yorkston, K. M., Beukelman, D. R., Strand, E. A., & Hakel, M. (2010). *Management of motor speech disorders in children and adults* (3rd ed.). Pro-Ed.

VOICE DISORDERS

Ma, E. P., Yiu, E. M., & Verdolini Abbott, K. (2007). Application of the ICF in voice disorders. *Seminars in Speech and Language, 28*(4), 343–350. https://DOI: 10.1055/s-2007-986531

LARYNGECTOMY

Cox, S. R., Theurer, J. A., Spaulding, S. J., & Doyle, P. C. (2015). The multidimensional impact of total laryngectomy on women. *Journal of Communication Disorders, 56,* 59–75. https://doi.org/10.1016/j.jcomdis.2015.06.008

Eadie, T. L. (2007). Application of the ICF in communication after total laryngectomy. *Seminars in Speech and Language, 28*(4), 291–300. https://DOI: 10.1055/s-2007-986526

HEARING IMPAIRMENT

Hickson L., & Scarinci, N. (2007). Older adults with acquired hearing impairment: Applying the ICF in rehabilitation. *Seminars in Speech and Language, 28*(4), 283–290. https://DOI: 10.1055/s-2007-986525

CHAPTER 2

Impact of Speaker-Related Factors on Intelligibility

Key Points:

- Impairment in any of the speech subsystems (respiration, phonation, resonation, articulation, and prosody) can contribute to reduced intelligibility.

- Typically, the subsystems work together and if there is reduced function in one, others may compensate during speech.

- In adults with reduced intelligibility, causes can include dysarthria, acquired apraxia of speech, and voice disorders resulting from various causes, including head and neck cancer.

- Face masks can negatively impact the visual and auditory signals listeners receive from speakers.

- Different types of face masks will be more effective for speech purposes depending on the needs of your client and their communication partners.

A person's ability to produce speech sounds that listeners can understand is a critical component of intelligibility. This chapter covers considerations related to the speaker that will allow you to better evaluate and manage reduced intelligibility in your clients. We know reduced intelligibility is commonly caused by difficulties in the articulatory system. Although impaired articulation can definitely reduce the listener's understanding, other subsystems associated with speech production may also contribute to reduced intelligibility. A breakdown into the speech subsystems, including respiration, phonation, resonation, articulation, and prosody/rate will allow you to consider all potential factors affecting intelligibility. Using this organization allows us to examine speech factors from the driving force of the respiratory system that lead to the movements of the vocal folds that create the sound source, which is shaped by valves and filters of the resonatory and articulatory systems into speech.

SPEECH SUBSYSTEMS AND EFFECT ON INTELLIGIBILITY

To truly determine which factors may reduce a client's intelligibility, we must first start with an understanding of the disorders that lead to this communication barrier. You will have a much clearer and more accurate plan for improving intelligibility if you can evaluate to determine the effect each subsystem has on speech production. While we may think first about the articulatory system when addressing intelligibility, we need to consider all subsystems, with treatment planned as more than just articulatory training when appropriate (Rosenbek, 1984). It's also important to remember that the subsystems may interact with each other (Weismer, 2007). For example, the respiratory system has a great deal of influence on how the phonatory system functions. Impaired voice production, normally created by the respiratory and phonatory systems, may cause issues with voicing of consonants shaped by the articulatory system. This book does not include an extensive discussion of the neurological or physiological reasons for all reduced intelligibility. A general overview of issues related directly to the speaker, including a table for organization by subsystem, will be provided for the following disorders that may cause reduced intelligibility:

- Dysarthria
- Acquired Apraxia of Speech
- Voice Disorders
  - Neurologic Etiology
  - Functional Etiology

□ Organic Etiology

□ Structural/Surgical Etiology Related to Head and Neck Cancer

INTELLIGIBILITY ISSUES RELATED TO SPEAKERS WITH DYSARTHRIA

Dysarthria is a collective name for a group of neurological disorders that impair speech subsystems (Duffy, 2019). The impairment results from damage or disease affecting the brain or nerves, which innervate muscles to move structures that result in speech production. According to Duffy (2019), dysarthria results in abnormal "strength, speed, range, steadiness, tone, or accuracy of movements required for breathing, phonatory, resonatory, articulatory, or prosodic aspects of speech production" (p. 4). Neuromuscular impairments refer to movement difficulties that are a result of neurological injury or disease. Weakness is one type of impairment that refers to a reduced ability to produce force (Clark, 2003). We may see evidence of paralysis (no movement) or paresis (reduced movement) that impact actions of the subsystems needed to produce clear speech. The subsystems will be impacted by the etiology and neurological impact of the client's disease or neural injury, so we do not want to assume the underlying impairment is always weakness. Other types of movement impairment that speakers with dysarthria can experience include incoordination, ataxia, and disorders of disrupted muscle tone, such as spasticity or rigidity (Clark, 2003). SLPs should have a thorough understanding of the client's etiology and how their movements are impacted (see Duffy (2019) for detailed information on dysarthria types, neuromuscular impairment, and underlying etiologies).

A general discussion of the subsystems will provide information on how impairment of each may reduce a speaker's intelligibility, as well as their ability to communicate in their daily life. Many publications on the topic of dysarthria cover the work originally created by Darley, Aronson, and Brown (1969a, 1969b). The purpose of their work was to create a classification system based on perceptual errors, which resulted in identification of the distinct dysarthria types. Their classification system of dysarthria allows us to view the subsystems and possible contributions of each to reduced intelligibility. The information in this section represents the body functions and structures levels in the World Health Organization's (WHO) framework, known as the International Classification of Functioning, Disability and Health or ICF (World Health Organization, 2001). The reduced intelligibility experienced by speakers represents the activity limitations mentioned in the ICF system. Table 2–1 (see p. 31) shows impairment in subsystems that may cause reduced intelligibility related to dysarthria.

Respiration

Speech breathing is a task that requires strength, coordination, and timing from the respiratory system. Dysarthria may occur with weak, uncoordinated movements, which can lead to a lack of respiratory drive and the breath control necessary to produce intelligible speech. It may be difficult for speakers with dysarthria to take in enough air to produce speech. In some cases, the forces generated may be of a high enough volume (i.e., amount) to produce speech, but not well controlled at the level of the respiratory system. In this case, a person may run out of air before producing a word or getting to the end of a phrase or sentence. Due to the various effects of the different dysarthria types, we can expect these speakers to sound quite different from each other (Duffy, 2019). The physical impairment (i.e., weakness, spasticity, incoordination) related to dysarthria can reveal itself in a variety of ways in different speakers. Table 2–1 illustrates how respiratory issues may cause a lack of control of loudness in speakers with dysarthria. However, the type and severity of dysarthria may dictate what we hear. Some speakers will have excessive, uncontrollable loudness if they cannot regulate the output of air from the respiratory system. Others may have reduced loudness due to lack of adequate breath support or proper valving to control where the air goes and how fast it moves. If a speaker either doesn't start with a large enough amount of air or isn't able to control how quickly the air leaves the respiratory system, we may hear short phrases or trailing sentences ("When are we going to the . . . ").

It is important to note here that speakers who are dealing with impairment in the respiratory system may use compensatory strategies in order to help listeners understand. This may involve using their respiratory system to overcome issues with the phonatory system. For example, in a speaker with hyperadducted vocal folds (too much closure), there may be a use of increased respiratory pressure in compensation. Or a speaker who has hypoadducted vocal folds (too little closure) may end up using more respiratory pressure in order to make up for the wasted air that moves too quickly through the more open glottis (opening between the vocal folds). This increased respiratory effort can be physically tiring for a client and may also result in them using increased, possibly unhealthy vocal effort.

Phonation

Because it is very difficult to separate the interaction of respiration and phonation, authors who describe the speech subsystems may combine them into the respiratory/phonatory system (Weismer, 2007). To dig deeper into intelligibility aspects related to the speaker, these subsystems are presented separately, but it is important to recall that there is a great deal of interaction between them, as previously described in the respiratory section. We can consider several aspects of vocal fold movement that may influence the phonation of a speaker with dysarthria. Phonation results from pulses of air moving through the glottis when the vocal fold covers are opening and closing (mucosal wave). Changes in pitch, loudness, and quality of voice are related to changes in movements of the larynx. First, the weakness, impaired tone, or incoordination of the muscles that move the laryngeal structures can affect the ability of the glottis to open or close. Lack of adequate vocal fold closure will cause a breathy sounding voice as it allows more air to escape during phonation. If there is a complete lack of closure, the vocal folds will not open and close effectively to produce voice (aphonia). If there is excessive vocal fold closure, the voice will sound harsh. Extreme closure may result in the voice barely being produced, which can sound strained or strangled. Second, abnormal vocal fold movements can affect how the voice sounds. Weak, slow vocal fold movements may cause pitch breaks, or a lack of pitch change for inflection (monotone). If vocal fold or laryngeal movements are larger than usual, the person may demonstrate excessive pitch changes. Aperiodicity in vocal fold vibration (regularity of successive cycles) may cause diplophonia, which listeners will hear as two different pitches being produced at the same time. This may happen if one vocal fold is vibrating more quickly than the other or if they vibrate out of sync. Lack of coordination between the respiratory and phonatory system may lead to audible inspiration (stridor) or breaks in phonation as the person runs out of respiratory support. Stridor could also result from inadequate opening of the vocal folds or from a structural deficit; therefore, the cause should be determined to manage it correctly. Short phrases with breaths in between are another sign that the person does not have adequate respiratory support and/or control. Excessive, abnormal laryngeal movements can also result in a perceived vocal tremor in some speakers with dysarthria.

Resonance

Movements of the velopharyngeal port involve two main structures and many muscles. The velum elevates to contact the posterior pharyngeal wall, which moves toward it. The lateral walls of the pharynx also contribute to closure of the port by coming to midline and contacting the velum and the posterior pharyngeal wall. The connection between these structures causes closure of the velopharyngeal port and separates the oral cavity from the nasal cavity. Separation of these structures causes the velopharyngeal port to open, which allows some nasality into speech. In dysarthria, weakness of the muscles that move these structures may result in lack of velopharyngeal port closure or lack of correct timing for closure, sometimes termed velopharyngeal incompetence (VPI). We may hear consonants produced by speakers with VPI as imprecise. Pressure consonants may be particularly affected as the air is not directed in the normal pathway for production, but is escaping through the open velopharyngeal port. In order to produce the pressure consonant /b/, we need to build up intraoral pressure. If the velum and pharyngeal walls are not in contact at the right time during that production, the airflow will escape through the nose and intraoral pressure will be weak. This can cause the consonant distortion we may hear, even though the articulatory system may be working correctly. If velopharyngeal dysfunction is present, all sounds, even vowels, may sound hypernasal. Any of these factors can lead to reduced intelligibility (Rong et al., 2016), even independent of the articulatory system. Yorkston and colleagues (2010) provide great insight into the interaction of hypernasality with the other subsystems of speech. These authors state that higher ratings of hypernasality will occur in speakers with articulatory errors that are severe. Also, listeners judging nasality may perceive less nasality with reduced loudness levels (related to respiratory drive). Listeners may perceive nasal emission when there is airflow through the nose during production of non-nasal consonants (Yorkston et al., 2010). This often occurs with hypernasality and is another result of velopharyngeal dysfunction. Some clients will have management for hypernasality that involves a pharyngeal flap surgery or use of prosthetic devices such as a palatal/pharyngeal obturator or palatal lift designed by a prosthodontist. These strategies may be useful in helping achieve better closure of the velopharyngeal port to reduce hypernasality. Sometimes, use of these strategies may cause too much closure or a lack of control of the structures that listeners may perceive as hyponasality. We may also hear hyponasality if excessive contractions or mistimed contractions occur in the velopharyngeal musculature. In order to compensate for nasality issues, some clients may attempt to have more precise production of speech sounds by using a more posterior position of the tongue. Although some sounds may be more accurately produced, this results in an abnormal resonance known as oral cul-de-sac resonance, a term often used to describe the speech of people who are deaf. The posterior tongue carriage then reshapes the voice, which reduces the loudness level and may sound muffled. If you think about a cul-de-sac in your neighborhood, it's the same concept. The sound gets into the oral cavity but then gets trapped by the posterior position of the tongue and can't move out effectively for normal projection of sounds.

Articulation

Impaired articulation is a primary reason for reduced intelligibility in many cases, which explains why much of the attention in the study of intelligibility has focused on this area. Impaired articulation contributes to reduced intelligibility in dysarthria, although of course, there can be a connection to the other subsystems of speech. The sound source, which originates in the respiratory and laryngeal systems moves through the resonating cavities and gets further shaped by the articulators into speech sounds. We have stationary articulators, such as the teeth, and articulators that move, such as the velum, lips, tongue, and jaw. Neurological injury or disease can compromise the movements of these structures. We may see weakness, slowness, incoordination, reduced range/rate of movement, and in some cases involuntary movements of the articulators. For example, Parkinson's disease, which reduces overall coordination and speed of movement, could decrease accuracy of articulator movements during speech. Cranial nerves provide innervation to these articulators, and neurological injury or disease may also affect these nerves. The facial nerve innervates the lips, the hypoglossal nerve innervates the tongue, and the mandibular branch of the trigeminal nerve innervates the jaw. Several cranial nerves, including the pharyngeal branch of the vagus nerve, are responsible for closure of the velopharyngeal port. We know dysarthria, by definition, impacts the speed, timing, and accuracy of movement. The articulators must have precise timing in relation to the other subsystems. The Darley, Aronson, and Brown (1969a; 1969b) classification system for dysarthria included imprecise articulation as a classic hallmark characteristic of all dysarthria types. Imprecise movements of the articulators result in frequent substitution errors in speakers with dysarthria, yet it is important to consider all other factors when we plan management.

We produce vowels by changing the size and shape of the oral cavity where the sound resonates. If a person has difficulty with timing, speed, coordination, or accuracy of movement of the articulators, this may restrict their ability to change the size and shape of the oral cavity to correctly produce vowels. As mentioned in the previous paragraph, it may compromise pressure consonants if the resonatory system does not allow enough intraoral pressure to produce them. Intraoral pressure could also be reduced by a poor lip seal. In discussing the production of connected speech, Weismer (2007) reminds us that one way of examining the goal of speech is the consideration of acoustic-perceptual performance. However, we want to keep in mind that what we hear perceptually may be the result of different motor acts. The concept of motor equivalence indicates that the same movement goal could be accomplished in more than one manner (Perrier & Fuchs, 2015). Listeners can understand us if we are speaking with our jaw moving freely or if we have our jaw in a fixed position because we have an object like a lollipop in our mouth. We alter the way our other structures move to compensate for the lack of jaw movement. Research has indicated that a speaker producing the vowel /u/ may do so differently across various repetitions of the sound (Perkell et al., 1995). This research indicated that speakers may use a trade-off of adjusting more tongue-body elevation along with lip protrusion. These two articulators may be used and adjusted differently to produce the same perceptual production of the /u/. Knowing about motor equivalence allows us to consider possible compensatory strategies if speakers are unable to reach certain articulatory targets due to movement deficits with articulators.

Prosody/Rate

Prosody reflects the coordinated effort of the other speech subsystems. Authors describing speech characteristics classify articulation as "segmental" and prosody as "suprasegmental" elements (Weismer, 2007; Yorkston et al., 2010). Prosody refers to the melody and rhythm of speech and consists of three principal features: stress patterning, intonation, and rate-rhythm (Yorkston et al., 2010). Stress in speech refers to emphasis placed on certain syllables or words. Speakers may use loudness, length of utterance (duration), and pitch changes as ways to mark stress. As stated in the earlier sections of this chapter, the other subsystems may cause the inability to control loudness, length of utterance, and pitch. This may result in disordered prosodic features in a speaker with dysarthria. A useful example of intonation occurs when our pitch inflection rises slightly at the end of a question, "Are you going to the store?" If you think about it, you have probably heard people ask you that question but using a statement format, such as, "You going to the store?" If a speaker produces the latter statement with a rising inflection or increased pitch toward the end, the listener would likely interpret it as a question. In this way, the inflection is as meaningful as the actual sentence structure. A speaker with dysarthria who has compromised respiratory and phonatory control may have difficulty controlling or changing inflection. Rate changes are prominent in speakers with dysarthria and may be the result of the inability to produce speech quickly. Changes in rate may be a compensatory measure used in order to help listeners understand more easily. In many cases, because of reduced speed, timing, and coordination of movement, rate will be slower in speakers with dysarthria compared to non-disordered speakers. One exception may occur in hypokinetic dysarthria, which results from Parkinson's disease, where some individuals demonstrate short, rapid rushes of speech (Duffy, 2019). It is important to consider that the overall concept of rate involves both how fast movements take place as well as the amount and placement of pauses that occur during speech. These will be important factors when you consider management strategies that may focus on rate. There are many resources and books written on the characteristics of the different dysarthria types. See Table 2–1 for a summary of the subsystems involved in clients with dysarthria and potential effects on intelligibility. For specific information on differential diagnosis and characteristics of all dysarthria types, please see Duffy (2019), Chapters 4 to 10, Weismer (2007), Chapter 1, and Yorkston et al. (2010), Chapter 3.

Table 2–1. Effect of Neuromotor Involvement on Intelligibility in Dysarthria

Subsystems	Impairment Resulting from Neuromotor Involvement Related to:	Effect on Speech Intelligibility
	Weakness	
	Spasticity	
	Incoordination	
Respiration	Reduced lung capacity	Excessive to reduced loudness
	Respiratory weakness	Short phrases
	Reduced respiratory support or control	Lack of air to finish sentences heard as a sentence that trails off
Phonation	Too tightly or too loosely closed vocal folds	Breathy to aphonic Harsh to strained/strangled
	Aperiodicity in vocal fold vibration	Diplophonia
	Slow, weak vocal fold movements	Pitch breaks
	Excessive vocal fold/laryngeal movements	Monotone to excessive pitch changes
	Lack of coordination between respiratory and phonatory systems	Stridor
		Phonation breaks
		Voice tremor
Resonance	Limited closure of the velopharyngeal port	Hypernasality Nasal emission
	Weak velar movement resulting in incoordination of the velopharyngeal port	Vowel and consonant distortions Cul-de-sac resonance Hyponasality
	Posterior positioning of the tongue	
Articulation	Weak, imprecise movements of the articulators, including the tongue, lips, and jaw	Imprecise consonants
		Substitution errors
		Weak pressure consonants
		Vowel distortion
Prosody/rate	All subsystem impairments listed above may contribute to issues with prosody and rate.	Reduced stress
		Equal and excess stress
		Monotone
		Monoloudness
		Short phrases with faster rate
		Slow rate

Sources: Duffy (2019); Weismer (2007).

INTELLIGIBILITY ISSUES RELATED TO SPEAKERS WITH ACQUIRED APRAXIA OF SPEECH

To most effectively manage treatment, it is important to differentiate between acquired apraxia of speech (AAOS) and other disorders. AAOS differs from dysarthria in that nonspeech actions of the speech muscles are often normal (e.g. tongue protrusion), indicating little/no weakness in AAOS. Dysarthria and/or aphasia can co-occur with AAOS, due to common etiologies. Duffy (2019) describes AAOS as

> a neurologic speech disorder that reflects an impaired capacity to plan or program sensorimotor commands necessary for directing movements that result in phonetically and prosodically normal speech. It can occur in the absence of physiologic disturbances associated with the dysarthrias and in the absence of disturbance in any component of language. (p. 269)

Rather than weakness, as associated with dysarthria, AAOS characteristics are related to impairment in the motor planning or programming required for correct execution of speech movements (Duffy, 2019). AAOS compromises patterns of movements that are normally automatic for speech. Speech contexts that require higher levels of planning/programming, such as longer, more complex utterances often present more issues for this compromised system. Highly overlearned or automatic speech acts do not place as much demand on planning/programming systems (Duffy, 2019). This explains why nonspeech acts, and even some very automatic speech acts, such as the response of "I'm fine" when someone asks, "How are you?" can result in normal movement and speech production. In the ICF classification system discussed in Chapter 1, the information in this section represents body functions and structure levels. Table 2–2 shows impairment in subsystems that may cause reduced intelligibility related to AAOS.

Respiration, Phonation, and Resonance

Because individuals with AAOS rarely experience difficulties related to breathing, phonating, or resonance (Duffy, 2019), this discussion will cover these subsystems as a group. Table 2–2 shows the individual breakdowns of the subsystems. Even though individually, these subsystems may not have strong impact, the lack of coordination and timing between respiration, phonation, and/or resonation may negatively affect speech production. To produce a sound source for speech, the respiratory system and phonatory system jointly coordinate movements of structures and air for vocal fold vibration. Studies of acoustic measures in individuals with AAOS

Table 2–2. Effect of Neuromotor Involvement on Intelligibility in Acquired Apraxia of Speech

Subsystems	Impairment Resulting from Planning/Programming Involvement Related to:	Effect on Speech Production
	Disturbed speech patterns Unorganized sequences of movements	
Respiration	Impaired sequencing and timing with phonatory system	Respiratory incoordination and timing issues may contribute to other speech effects listed in this table.
Phonation	Laryngeal and supralaryngeal articulatory variability in movements	There may not be accurate differentiation between voiced and voiceless stops and fricatives.
Resonance	Timing issues with velar movements in relation to articulation and phonation	Inconsistent hypernasality Inconsistent hyponasality
Articulation and fluency	Issues with sequencing, timing, and coordination of the articulators, including the tongue, lips, velum, and jaw	Consonant and vowel distortions Distortions include: ■ Substitutions ■ Additions ■ Repetitions ■ Sound prolongations Increased errors with length and complexity Trial and error groping behaviors False articulatory starts
Prosody/rate	All subsystem impairments listed above may contribute to issues with prosody and rate, which are often very noticeable in acquired apraxia of speech.	Slow rate Equal stress or stress errors Increased pauses within utterances

Source: Duffy (2019).

have demonstrated differences in voice onset time (VOT) and airflow during fricative production (Duffy, 2019). VOT can be defined as the time between the burst in a plosive sound and the initiation of the next voiced phoneme (Caruso & Klasner Burton, 1987). VOT may be useful as an acoustic measure, as it shows timing between the respiratory-laryngeal systems in relation to the articulatory-resonatory systems. Ziegler and von Cramon (1986) found timing impairment of velar movement in individuals with AAOS in relationship to articulation and phonation. Issues related to timing of velar movements may result in hyper or hypo-nasality, as the resonatory system may not interact in sync with the other subsystems. The clinical take-home point from these acoustic measures is that the lack of coordinated movements between respiratory, phonatory, and resonatory systems can reduce intelligibility. These subsystems can be examined independently, but their interaction should also be considered.

Articulation and Fluency

Individuals with AAOS frequently report that articulation is a major area of concern (Duffy, 2019). Unlike dysarthria, where weakness or paralysis interferes with articulatory movements and precision, the sequencing, timing, and coordination of these movements are affected in AAOS. Sound distortions, such as substitutions and omissions, as well as sound repetitions and prolongations, occur frequently. AAOS can reduce fluency as these repetitions and prolongations interrupt continuous flows of speech. False articulatory starts to words and sentences further compromise fluency. A classic characteristic of AAOS is the groping trial and error productions as the individual attempts to correctly produce speech targets. Longer and more complex utterances that require more planning and programming skills will be more affected than shorter or more automatic speech tasks (Duffy, 2019). We may see this when the person can produce the word "but" but then demonstrate increasing error with longer words like "butter" or "butterfly."

Prosody and Rate

Interference with planning and sequencing of movements across the subsystems combine to significantly impair prosody in speakers with AAOS. Jacks (2009) reported on several previous investigations that articulatory precision and syllable segregation (i.e., each syllable is produced in isolation from the next) are major contributory factors in prosodic impairment in AAOS. The syllable segregation and equal stress patterns across both stressed and unstressed syllables further reduces normal prosody. In speakers with AAOS, overall rate of speech is slow, with excessive prolongation of consonant and vowel sounds (Duffy, 2019). Table 2–2 provides a summary of subsystems affected by AAOS and possible involvement on intelligibility. To find specific, detailed information on acquired apraxia of speech, please refer to the following chapters: Duffy (2019), Chapter 11, Yorkston et al. (2010), Chapter 12.

INTELLIGIBILITY ISSUES RELATED TO SPEAKERS WITH VOICE DISORDERS

When we think about reduced intelligibility, most of us probably consider articulation to be the major contributing factor. Voice disorders or dysphonia may not be something that you've considered could reduce intelligibility in a significant way. Impairment in any of the three subsystems that allow us to produce voice (respiratory, phonatory, and resonatory) can, in fact, reduce a person's intelligibility. Loudness, pitch, and quality are three parameters of voice that could reduce intelligibility. Loudness makes a difference in helping us to understand a speaker's message (Ramig, 1992). A voice that is not loud enough will be difficult to understand, so it is important to consider if loudness is reducing a speaker's intelligibility. A speaker's pitch may also influence how easily listeners can understand. One way this can occur is through inflection. If inflection is missing, the lack of prosody may reduce a speaker's intelligibility (De Bodt et al., 2002). A study by Rong and colleagues (2016) examined individuals with speech and voice disorders secondary to ALS and found that the largest contributing subsystem to decreased intelligibility was the articulatory system, followed by the resonatory system, and phonatory systems. This research informs us that voice quality factors, such as breathiness, harshness, or hypernasality may reduce intelligibility. Studies have shown that individuals who have voice disorders, yet normal articulation, have reduced intelligibility compared to speakers with normal voices (Evitts et al., 2016; Porcaro et al., 2019). Due to the variability of causes and influence of voice disorders, our discussion of voice will be organized by different etiologies. It is critical for SLPs working with clients who have voice disorders to have regular contact with medical professionals. These individuals may include otolaryngologists (ENTs), neurologists, and gastroenterologists. The SLP can monitor progress by measuring perceptual or acoustical changes in voice production. However, a disordered voice will frequently occur along with a medical diagnosis (e.g., Parkinson's disease or vocal nodules) and SLPs may work with other professionals to monitor progress in all areas related to voice production.

Voice Disorders Related to Neurologic Etiology

Some voice disorders result from damage or disease that limits functioning of the neurological systems providing innervation related to voice production. This might involve conditions that impact functioning in the central nervous system, which includes the brain and spinal cord. For our purposes regarding the central nervous system, we will focus on the cerebral cortex, cerebellum, and basal ganglia as the primary neural areas (substrates) that help us produce voice. The peripheral nervous system that contributes to voice production involves mainly the cranial nerves that innervate laryngeal, velopharyngeal, and oral structures. One spinal nerve, the phrenic nerve, is responsible for innervation of the diaphragm, which is one of the most important muscles of respiration. There is a great deal of overlap between neurogenic dysphonia and dysarthria, because both have the potential to affect voice due to neurological issues. If you are working with a client who has neurogenic dysphonia, further reading on this topic would be helpful. For specific information on neurogenic voice disorders, please see Boone et al. (2019), Chapter 5 or Sapienza and Hoffman (2022), Chapter 6. Resources listed in the previous section of this chapter on dysarthria will also provide specific details on neurogenic dysphonia.

Voice Disorders Related to Functional Etiology

Boone and colleagues (2019) describe functional voice disorders as occurring when the respiration, phonation, and resonation systems appear capable of producing a non-disordered voice, but there is not a proper functional balance between the subsystems to produce normal voice. Basically, the cause of dysphonia with a functional etiology is the way the person uses their voice. Muscle tension dysphonia (MTD) is the most common voice disorder in both children and adults (Boone et al., 2019). Excessive tension or voice use can cause a disordered voice itself but may also result in formation of vocal masses like nodules or polyps. We may see clients who have developed poor vocal hygiene habits, such as coughing, throat clearing, smoking, and not hydrating enough. Any of these factors play a role in how the voice sounds and could influence the person's intelligibility. See Table 2–3 for information about typical functional voice disorders, including characteristics and the potential effect of each on intelligibility. For more information on causes, symptoms, and treatment of functional voice disorders, please see Boone et al. (2019), Chapter 3 or Sapienza and Hoffman (2022), Chapter 5.

Voice Disorders Related to Organic Etiology

Boone and colleagues (2019) define organic voice disorders as those "related to structural deviations of the vocal tract (lungs, muscles of respiration, larynx, pharynx, and oral cavity) or to diseases of specific structures of the vocal tract" (p. 11). Whereas Sapienza and Hoffman (2022) acknowledge the classifications of "functional," "organic," and "neurogenic," these

Table 2–3. Characteristics Affecting Intelligibility in Functional Voice Disorders

Functional Voice Disorder	Characteristics	Effect on Intelligibility
Vocal fold nodules	Bilateral growths that vary in size and texture Start off as blistery growths, but over time may develop a harder texture like a callous Most frequently caused by phonotrauma/vocal abuse	Breathiness Reduced loudness Lower pitch Worsens with voice usage
Vocal fold polyps	Usually unilateral growths May be bilateral or multiple Small and broad-based (sessile) but some grow on a small stalk (pedunculated) Causes include phonotrauma/vocal abuse, smoking, allergies	Breathiness Reduced loudness Diplophonia (if not symmetrical) Vocal fatigue
Reinke's edema or generalized edema	Swelling due to accumulation of fluid in the vocal folds, usually bilateral High incidence in smokers	Low pitch Gravelly (smoker's voice)
Laryngitis	Acute: related to pneumonia or upper respiratory illness and very common Chronic: less common, long lasting version of acute Traumatic: related to excessive or strained phonation	Breathiness Harsh or strained Low pitch Possible aphonia

Sources: Boone et al. (2019); Sapienza and Hoffman (2022).

authors organized their textbook to cover both functional and organic disorders under a more general category of "vocal pathology." This system can be useful in recognizing that there is a relationship between functional and organic dysphonia. Although we might like to put voice disorders neatly into categories related to cause, there are often overlapping factors related to both functional and organic etiologies. For example, people may develop vocal nodules mainly through the way they use their voice. This person may use excessive muscular tension, yell, smoke, or use hard glottal attacks, which represent functional causes. By the time a doctor has diagnosed nodules, a structural deviation or lesion has developed.

Another example might be a person who begins with a structural deviation, such as contact ulcers related to Gastroesophageal Reflux Disease (GERD) who reacts to the hoarseness and breathiness in their voice by speaking with more tension. What began as an organic disorder (GERD) is influenced by the way the person uses their voice, bringing in functional factors as well. Following the organizational system in Boone et al. (2019), Table 2–4 describes typical organic voice disorders, common characteristics of each, and the potential factors related to intelligibility. Use of the term "hoarse" is controversial among some voice professionals. According to Stachler and colleagues (2018), many clinicians and physicians incorrectly use hoarseness and dysphonia interchangeably. These authors suggest that hoarseness is a symptom reported by patients of altered voice quality and dysphonia defines impaired voice production as noted by a clinician. For a review of terms used to describe voice, you can find detailed information in Boone et al. (2019), Chapter 4, and Sapienza and Hoffman (2022), Chapter 5.

Voice Disorders Related to Head and Neck Cancer

Head and Neck (H&N) cancer is another medical diagnosis that will have a significant effect on a person's voice and ability to be understood. Changes in communication abilities following laryngectomy may cause social isolation (Danker et al., 2010) and can significantly impact a person's quality of life (Vilaseca et al., 2006) and overall level of communication participation (Eadie et al., 2016). Although hearing the term H&N cancer may cause us to think mainly of laryngeal cancer, there are many lesion sites that could affect voice and/or speech including: oral cavity, pharynx, nasal cavity, larynx, salivary glands, ear, neck (Sapienza & Hoffman, 2022). We know that individuals with voice disorders may have great variability within and between speakers, and this is also true of alaryngeal speakers. To have a better understanding of the types of intelligibility impairment these clients may encounter, it is important for us to understand the treatment types and how they may affect the tissues involved in producing voice as well.

Influence of Head and Neck Cancer Treatment on Voice

Following a diagnosis of H&N cancer, members of the medical team will work together to manage the patient's treatment. Options may include surgery, radiation therapy, chemoradiation (combination of chemotherapy and radiation therapy). These may occur in isolation or in combination, depending on the medical needs of the patient. According to Sapienza and Hoffman (2022), chemotherapy is not used to cure H&N cancer in isolation. There are many studies comparing the influence of these different

Table 2-4. Characteristics Affecting Intelligibility in Organic Voice Disorders

Organic Voice Disorder	Characteristics	Effect on Intelligibility
Acid reflux disease	Gastroesophageal Reflux Disease (GERD): stomach acid moves from the stomach into the esophagus Laryngopharyngeal Reflux Disease (LPRD): stomach acid moves from stomach through upper esophageal sphincter and may contact the laryngeal structures, including vocal folds	Perceived voice changes, particularly in the morning (related to increased movement of acid during the night)
Contact ulcers and granulomas	Contact ulcers: small sores that form on the vocal folds due to irritation Granuloma: larger mass lesion when granulated tissue grows over the contact ulcer Causes of contact ulcers/granuloma: (1) Excessive slamming of vocal folds and use of hard glottal attacks (functional cause) (2) Untreated LPRD due to acid irritation of vocal folds (organic cause) (3) Intubation trauma may occur when a patient in intubated or extubated for surgery	Roughness Low pitch These symptoms may become more severe with granuloma as they are a larger mass lesion which may reduce vocal fold closure and movement more than contact ulcers.
Laryngeal cysts	Usually unilateral Causes: (1) Blocked duct of mucous glands (2) Phonotrauma/vocal abuse	Perceived voice changes

continues

39

Table 2–4. *continued*

Organic Voice Disorder	Characteristics	Effect on Intelligibility
Recurrent respiratory papillomatosis	Wart-like growths mainly caused by human papilloma virus (HPV) that can occur in the trachea, larynx, pharynx, oral cavity, velum, etc.	Roughness Breathiness Shortness of breath Stridor Low pitch
Sulcus vocalis	Reflux or phonotrauma/vocal abuse may be the cause. Indentation in tissue, usually bilateral and symmetrical	Strained Reduced loudness Monotone Aphonia
Laryngeal web	Webbing that grows between the vocal folds prevents normal movement. Congenital: the membrane between the vocal folds does not separate during fetal development Acquired: following bilateral trauma to the medial edges of the vocal folds, healing may result in the folds growing together	Shortness of breath Stridor High pitch

Sources: Boone et al. (2019); Sapienza and Hoffman (2022).

treatments on voice in H&N cancer patients. This chapter will cover only general results because the usefulness to our topic of intelligibility is not so much whether one treatment is more beneficial than another. It is more important for us to consider whether, in addition to voice symptoms related to the cancer itself, the treatment can also negatively affect the voice. Post-radiation voice symptoms can include hoarseness, changes in pitch, loudness, or quality (Sapienza & Hoffman, 2022). There is also often a thickening of mucus, which may lead to more throat clearing and coughing, putting the vocal folds through further trauma. Bibby and colleagues (2008) reported that post-chemoradiation therapy resulted in breathy, strained, and rough voices. As an additional concern, our bodies need proper hydration to provide adequate lubrication to the laryngeal system, and chemoradiation dries the mucosal tissues and can cause muscle atrophy (Lazarus, 2009).

Depending on many factors, including the size, location, and stage of the H&N tumor, doctors consider different surgeries. There are options that do not involve a total removal of the larynx, which may leave enough structural tissue intact for the client to phonate, known as conservation surgery. Even clients who undergo this type of treatment will probably have disordered voices and reduced intelligibility, although results may be better than for those who undergo a total laryngectomy. It is beyond this book to discuss the different surgeries and how each might affect voice. You can find a useful overview of several surgical options in the research of Crosetti and colleagues (2017), who examined alaryngeal speakers following multiple types of treatment for laryngeal cancer. Their findings showed intelligibility ranged from mild to severe in patients who experienced all types of surgeries, including conservation. In participants who had vocal folds left intact, breathiness and damage to the vocal folds resulted in impaired voice quality. There are many variations of medical treatment in patients who undergo conversion surgery for H&N cancer, so they are a very heterogeneous group. Voice quality will vary based on the procedure, structures removed, and tissue remaining for phonatory purposes.

Clients who have a laryngectomy will need to rely on alaryngeal options for communication. The larynx and vocal folds have been surgically removed and traditional phonation is no longer possible. It is important to remember that these individuals may have also had treatment in the form of radiation or chemotherapy. Options for alaryngeal speech include the use of electrolaryngeal (EL), esophageal speech (ES), and tracheoesophageal (TE) speech. These options and some of their pros and cons related to intelligibility are discussed below.

Electrolaryngeal Speech

Individuals can use an artificial larynx in two different ways to produce EL speech. The first involves placement of the device on the neck or cheek. The artificial larynx is a mechanical device that creates a buzzing sound by vibrating a diaphragm. This buzzing sound takes the place of the sound source that the person previously created using vocal fold vibrations. This pulsed sound vibration moves through the neck or cheek into the oral cavity and then the articulators shape the buzzing sound source into speech sounds. Figure 2–1 illustrates placement of an artificial larynx used to produce EL speech in this manner.

Some individuals cannot produce an adequate sound source for speech, usually related to hard, fibrotic tissue resulting from medical treatment. The sound source may not be able to penetrate through tissues into the oral cavity. In this case, a small plastic tube is mounted onto

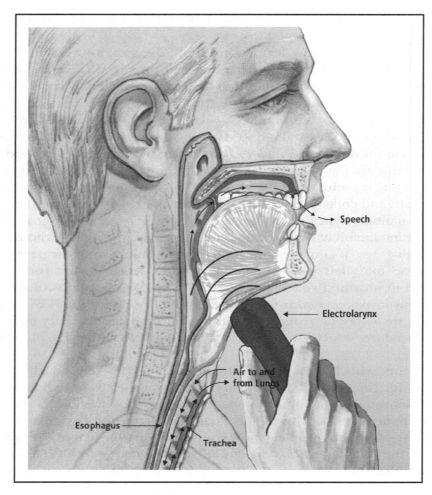

Figure 2–1. Optimal placement of electrolarynx. Copyright © 2017 Anatomical Training Aid. Reprinted by permission of InHealth Technologies (a business of Freudenberg Medical, LLC).

the same device and the individual inserts the intraoral device into their mouth. Figure 2–2 illustrates an electrolarynx that is fitted with this intra-oral adapter. The device creates a buzzing sound source that the tube carries into the oral cavity for the articulators to shape into speech. Clients often use an artificial larynx early on, as it is fairly easy to use right after surgery. EL speech serves as a primary communication method for some individuals, and others use it as a backup method when there is difficulty using another method.

There is wide variability in intelligibility levels in EL research, partly based on the speaker's performance using the device (Rothman, 1978). Speakers rated with better intelligibility turned their EL on and off at the correct times and maintained a steady contact with the device on their neck. Cox (2019) published an excellent article reviewing the use of EL speech, summarizing several studies of EL speech and reported intelligibility ranges from 16% to 90%. In general, EL speakers obtained lower intelligibility scores compared to ES and TE speakers (Hillman et al., 1998; van Sluis et al., 2018). However, Clark and Stemple (1982) reported that in background noise, EL speakers were more intelligible than other alaryngeal speakers. It is important to note that EL speakers indicated poor/

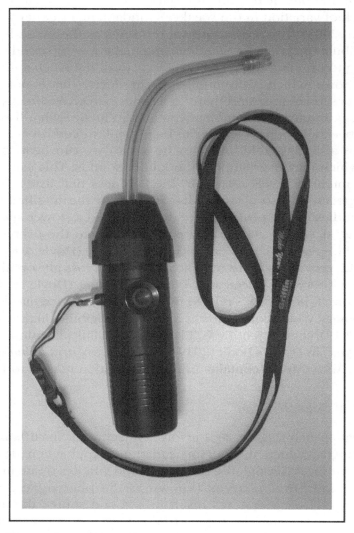

Figure 2–2. Electrolarynx fitted with intraoral adapter. From *Voice Disorders, Fourth Edition* (p. 337) by Christine Sapienza and Bari Hoffman. Copyright © 2022 Plural Publishing, Inc. All rights reserved.

fair voice-related quality of life because of difficulty being understood in noise or on the phone (Cox & Doyle, 2014).

EL speech has unique characteristics, and "robotic" is a common term used to describe it. Doyle and Eadie (2005) report this quality as unnatural and mechanical sounding to listeners. We could also describe EL speech as monotone, as the speaker can often set a "high" versus "low" pitch, but inflection-type variation has not been possible until recently and may not be accessible to all users. Some devices now have a dial that the speaker can raise or lower to adjust the pitch, but this requires a fair amount of skill. The monotone quality and mechanical nature of the voice may result from a lack of variation in the speaker's fundamental frequency (Meltzner & Hillman, 2005). This monotone speech reduces the prosodic elements that contribute to speech intelligibility and make speech sound natural and interesting to listeners (Bien et al., 2008). Part of the mechanical nature is radiating noise, which is the hum from the device that is not filtered by the speaker's vocal tract and that the listener perceives directly (Saikachi et al., 2009). Intensity or loudness can also influence what listeners hear with EL speech. Loudness levels can be difficult to control as the settings on devices are adjustable but must be set so we can hear the quietest sounds, which may over-amplify the louder sounds. This can cause variability in intensity levels related to the loudness that listeners perceive. Rate of speech is also a factor that influences the intelligibility of EL speech. Studies of EL speakers have demonstrated a slower speaking rate (Hillman et al., 1998), which may partly be due to the over-articulation that most EL speakers use to enhance intelligibility (Doyle & Eadie, 2005). Using an EL provides a constant voicing source across all sounds, so there is no contrast between voiced and voiceless cognates (Doyle et al., 1988). A combination of these issues related to use of an EL device may be distracting to listeners, which could further reduce intelligibility in these speakers. Nagle's (2019) chapter entitled, "Elements of Clinical Training with the Electrolarynx" in Doyle's book (2019), *Clinical Care and Rehabilitation in Head and Neck Cancer* contains useful information related to EL speech.

Esophageal Speech

Esophageal speech (Figure 2–3) involves injecting or insufflating air into the esophagus, which the person can then expel when desired. The expelled air moves through the esophagus and vibrates tissue in the upper esophagus and lower pharynx (known as the pharyngoesophageal or PE segment). These vibrations result in a sound source the articulators can shape into speech (Diedrich, 1968). There are many reasons that individuals value ES over, or in addition to, other methods of alaryngeal communication. One reason is that this method is free of cost. Doyle and Finchem (2019) mention reduced potential for aspiration due to the lack of a tracheostomy fistula and possible improved pitch and loudness control

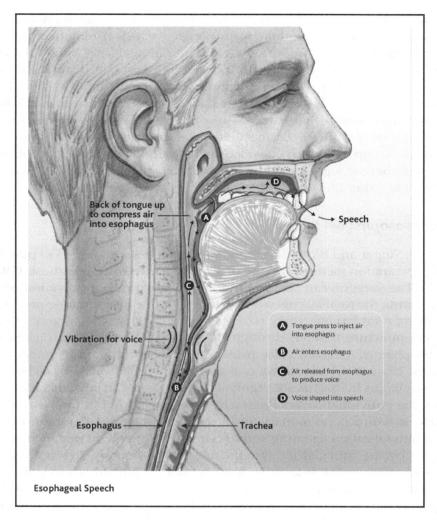

Back of tongue up to compress air into esophagus

A

Speech

D

Vibration for voice

C

B

A Tongue press to inject air into esophagus

B Air enters esophagus

C Air released from esophagus to produce voice

D Voice shaped into speech

Esophagus

Trachea

Esophageal Speech

Figure 2–3. Production of esophageal speech. Copyright © 2017 Anatomical Training Aid. Reprinted by permission of InHealth Technologies (a business of Freudenberg Medical, LLC).

as benefits of ES. For detailed instructions on how to facilitate the use of ES with clients, please see the excellent chapter by Doyle and Finchem (2019) entitled, "Teaching Esophageal Speech: A Process of Collaborative Instruction" found in the book edited by Doyle (2019), *Clinical Care and Rehabilitation in Head and Neck Cancer.*

The effect of ES on intelligibility will vary between different speakers, who may be more or less proficient in its use. Researchers over the years have reported that ES is characterized by a rough and breathy voice (Clark & Stemple, 1982) with limited loudness (Max et al., 1996) and low pitch

(Snidecor & Curry, 1959). Salmon (2005) further noted that many individuals using ES may only produce short phrases, which could affect intelligibility. Weinberg (1983) reported a slow rate in speakers using ES. Doyle and Finchem (2019) also mention behaviors that might distract listeners, including "stoma blast" when noise occurs when air moves through the stoma, as well as facial grimacing or noticeable neck tension. In addition, research has shown that listeners use different eye-gaze patterns when communicating with an alaryngeal speaker, particularly one who uses ES (Evitts & Gallop, 2011). In considering any of these factors, it is critical to note that there is a great deal of variability as some individuals are highly intelligible using ES while others are not as successful.

Tracheoesophageal Speech

In 1979, Singer and Blom developed the tracheoesophageal (TE) puncture voice restoration method and the first TE puncture voice prosthesis (Blom, 1998). The surgeon can perform the TE puncture voice restoration procedure during the total laryngectomy surgery, or during a separate procedure following total laryngectomy (Gress & Singer, 2005). The surgeon creates a small puncture (fistula) through the posterior wall of the trachea into the esophagus. A valved voice prosthesis is inserted into this puncture to prevent closure, which allows one-way flow of air from the trachea into the esophagus below the PE segment (Figure 2–4). During exhalation, and when the individual covers the tracheostoma with their thumb or another device, it redirects pulmonary air into the esophagus, setting the PE segment into vibration, creating sound (Gress & Singer, 2005), which is then shaped by the articulatory system into speech sounds. Research shows that use of TE speech is fairly simple and fast for individuals to learn, with a success rate reported between 80% to 90% (Blom et al., 1986; Gress & Singer, 2005). TE speech is pulmonary driven, meaning air from lungs is used to vibrate the PE segment, and thus more closely resembles typical, laryngeal speech than either ES or EL. Because the air supply comes from the lungs, TE speech may lead to longer phonation time and higher intelligibility ratings compared to ES and EL speech (Doyle et al., 1988).

Like other forms of alaryngeal speech, the use of TE speech will differ based on the anatomy and skill of the user. Some listeners may prefer TS over ES or EL (Sapienza & Hoffman, 2022) but not surprisingly, it has been rated more poorly by listeners than laryngeal speech (Williams & Watson, 1987; van As et al., 2003). Challenges to the voice and speech intelligibility with TE speech can include pitch, which is the same lower pitch for both females and males (Trudeau & Qi, 1990). Theoretically, all sounds are voiced with TE speech, therefore, voice/voiceless distinctions are not clear to listeners. However, studies found that some individuals using TE speech can produce voiceless sounds and are even able to

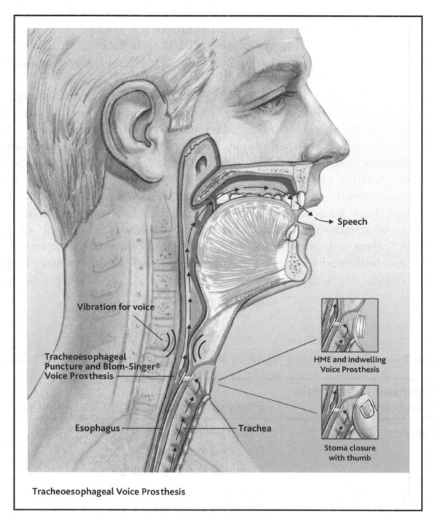

Figure 2–4. Production of speech utilizing tracheoesophageal voice prosthesis. Copyright © 2017 Anatomical Training Aid. Reprinted by permission of InHealth Technologies (a business of Freudenberg Medical, LLC).

whisper (Doyle et al., 1988; Searl, 2017). In some TE speech users, listeners may perceive a wet sounding voice, likely because of pharyngeal secretions (Blom et al., 1986) and the voice could be characterized as tight or breathy, depending upon the user's skill (Eadie & Doyle, 2004). Rate of speech in individuals using TE speech can fall into normal to slower than normal ranges (Blom et al., 1986). The variability of TE devices and users makes it difficult to classify voices of individuals who use TE speech as a homogeneous group. For further information on the options and use of TE devices, please see Graville et al.'s (2019) chapter entitled, "Voice Restoration with the Tracheoesophageal Voice Prosthesis: The Current State of the Art" in Doyle (2019).

In considering challenges to intelligibility in the individuals who have undergone H&N cancer, there are multiple variables and factors, even within just one of the methods of alaryngeal communication. For this reason, a careful evaluation of specific aspects related to each speaker will be vitally important. In order to work effectively with these clients, SLPs may need further education and hands-on training. Lastly, SLPs should educate individuals who require alaryngeal speech methods on all options and allow them to select what works best. Table 2–5 summarizes both the effect of treatment options and types of alaryngeal speech on intelligibility. For more complete information on head and neck cancer, please see books dedicated to the topic, including Casper and Colton (1998) or Doyle (2019).

Table 2–5. Characteristics Affecting Intelligibility in Head and Neck Cancer

Management Related to H&N Cancer	Effect on Voice Related to Intelligibility
Radiation	Pitch changes
	Reduced loudness
	Changes in voice quality
Chemoradiation	Breathiness
	Strain
	Roughness
Conservation surgery, partial laryngectomy	Breathiness
	Reduced loudness control
	Reduced pitch control
	Large variability based on procedure and tissue removal
Electrolaryngeal (EL) speech	Monotone
	Monoloudness to extreme variability in loudness
	Unnatural sounding
	Mechanical sounding (radiating noise)
	Lack of voice/voiceless contrasts

Table 2–5. *continued*

Management Related to H&N Cancer	Effect on Voice Related to Intelligibility
Esophageal speech (ES)	Roughness
	Breathiness
	Low pitch
	Reduced loudness
	Short phrases
	Slow rate
	Lack of voice/voiceless contrasts
Tracheoesophageal (TE) speech	Breathiness
	Tight voice
	Low pitch
	Slow rate
	Lack of voice/voiceless contrasts

Sources: Doyle (2019); Sapienza and Hoffman (2022).

EFFECT OF FACE MASKS AND SOCIAL DISTANCING ON INTELLIGIBILITY

To stay safe during the pandemic, people learned to communicate differently and some of the changes to our usual face-to-face style affected intelligibility. Face masks have been shown to limit the acoustic signal, especially on high frequencies that provide listeners with important information (Corey et al., 2020; Vos et al., 2021). A study by Corey and colleagues (2020) examined how much listeners could understand from a non-disordered speaker using 12 different masks. Their results indicated that blue surgical masks provided the best acoustic information to listeners and that adding layers to masks reduces acoustic information. To provide the missing visual information during speech sessions, clinicians may use a clear shield or mask with a clear window in the mouth area. Corey and colleagues (2020) found that these types of masks negatively affected acoustic information more than other types of masks and that reflection or fogging of the mask can also interfere with visual information for listeners.

Whereas a speaker who does not have reduced intelligibility may be able to easily compensate for the compromised acoustic signals with masks by speaking more loudly, wearing a mask may require additional effort on the part of a speaker with reduced intelligibility. Socially distancing involves keeping more distance between speakers and listeners, which will likely require extra effort and attention on the part of both to communicate effectively. Both masks and increased distance may reduce the visual information available to listeners, which can reduce intelligibility. If you are working with clients or family members who are socially distancing or wearing masks, these factors should be considered during your evaluation and management process, and suggestions will be made in upcoming chapters on these topics.

SUMMARY

Intelligibility can be reduced by disorders that impact speech and/or voice production. To fully examine the factors that impact a client's intelligibility, SLPs should consider all of the speech subsystems, including respiration, phonation, resonance, articulation, and prosody. These subsystems can impact intelligibility independently or in combination. Understanding the etiologies and how each of these subsystems is affected will allow SLPs to better address each client's individual challenges. Having knowledge about the impact of different types of face masks will help SLPs make the best suggestions to their clients about which masks to use. This increased understanding can lead to more effective evaluation and management of clients with reduced intelligibility.

 # Case Study

Dysarthria Case: Jack is a 22-year-old college student who sustained a TBI in the past year due to a fall, which resulted in a coma lasting for ten days. Following nine months of rehabilitative therapy, he was living at home while taking courses at a local university. His impairments included muscular weakness in the respiratory, phonatory, resonatory, and articulatory systems. Jack's reduced intelligibility limited his activities, as people outside of his immediate family had difficulty understanding him at times. Jack was not as active as he once was due to difficulty with communication. The restriction of Jack's participation included difficulties communicating in the classroom and in other campus activities.

Case Study

Voice Disorders Case: Beth is a 74-year-old female, living with her husband, adult daughter, and two young grandchildren. She and her family lived in a rural area, with a two-hour drive to the closest facility where she could receive voice services. During her ENT evaluation, Beth completed a written case history form indicating that she was not able to be loud enough to be heard in nearly all situations. Beth described her voice quality as rough and mentioned that people outside of her family could not understand everything she said and they often asked her to repeat herself, especially in noisy places. At times, even her family members had difficulty understanding her. She reported vocal fatigue when she participated in her usual activities, which included reading to her grandchildren, playing bridge with friends, and singing in her church choir. Because of the fatigue and voice breaks, she stopped most of her social activities and the restriction of her ability to be understood combined with vocal fatigue limited her typical participation socially and at home.

REFERENCES

Bibby, J. R., Cotton, S. M., Perry, A., & Corry, J. F. (2008). Voice outcomes after radiotherapy treatment for early glottic cancer: Assessment using multidimensional tools. *Head & Neck, 30*(5), 600–610. https://doi.org/10.1002/hed.20750

Bien, S., Rinaldo, A., Silver, C. E., Fagan, J. J., Pratt, L. W., Tarnowska, C., . . . Ferlito, A. (2008). History of voice rehabilitation following laryngectomy. *The Laryngoscope, 118*(3), 453–458. https://doi.org/10.1097/MLG.0b013e31815db4a2

Blom, E. D. (1998). Evolution of tracheoesophageal voice prostheses. In Blom, E. D., Singer, M. I., & Hamaker, R. C. (Eds.), *Tracheoesophageal voice restoration following total laryngectomy* (pp. 1–8). Singular Publishing Group.

Blom, E. D., Singer, M. I., & Hamaker, R. C. (1986). A prospective study of tracheoesophageal speech. *Archives of Otolaryngology—Head and Neck Surgery, 112*(4), 440–447. https://doi.org/10.1001/archotol.1986.03780040080017

Boone, D. R., McFarlane, S. C., Von Berg, S. L., & Zraick, R. I. (2019). *The voice and voice therapy* (10th ed.). Pearson.

Caruso, A., & Klasner Burton, E. (1987). Temporal acoustic measures of dysarthria associated with amyotrophic lateral sclerosis. *Journal of Speech-Language-Hearing Research, 30*, 80–87. https://doi.org/10.1044/jshr.3001.80

Casper, J. K., & Colton, R. H. (1998). *Clinical manual for laryngectomy and head/neck cancer rehabilitation* (2nd ed.). Singular Publishing Group.

Clark, H. M. (2003). Neuromuscular treatments for speech and swallowing: A tutorial. *American Journal of Speech-Language Pathology, 12*(4), 400–415. https://doi.org/10.1044/1058-0360(2003/086)

Clark, J. G., & Stemple, J. C. (1982). Assessment of three modes of alaryngeal speech with a synthetic sentence identification (SSI) task in varying message-to-competition ratios. *Journal of Speech and Hearing Research, 25*(3), 333–338. https://pubs.asha.org/doi/10.1044/jshr.2503.333

Corey, R. M., Jones, U., & Singer, A. C. (2020). Acoustic effects of medical, cloth, and transparent face masks on speech signals. *The Journal of the Acoustical Society of America, 148*(4), 2371–2375. https://doi.org/10.1121/10.0002279

Cox, S. R. (2019). Review of the electrolarynx: The past and present. *Perspectives of the ASHA Special Interest Groups, 4*(1), 118–129. https://doi.org/10.1044/2018_PERS-SIG3-2018-0013

Cox, S. R., & Doyle, P. C. (2014). The influence of electrolarynx use on postlaryngectomy voice-related quality of life. *Otolaryngology-Head & Neck Surgery, 150*(6), 1005–1009. https://doi.org/10.1177%2F0194599814524704

Crosetti, E., Fantini, M., Arrigoni, G., Salonia, L., Lombardo, A., Atzori, A., . . . Succo, G.. (2017). Telephonic voice intelligibility after laryngeal cancer treatment: Is therapeutic approach significant? *European Archives of Oto-Rhino-Laryngology, 274*, 337–346. https://doi.org/10.1007/s00405-016-4217-9

Danker, H., Wollbrück, D., Singer, S., Fuchs, M., Brähler, E., & Meyer, A. (2010). Social withdrawal after laryngectomy. *European Archives of Oto-Rhino-Laryngology, 267*, 593–600. https://doi.org/10.1007/s00405-009-1087-4

Darley, F. L., Aronson, A. E., & Brown, J. R. (1969a). Clusters of deviant speech dimensions in the dysarthrias. *Journal of Speech and Hearing Research, 12*(3), 462–496. https://doi.org/10.1044/jshr.1203.462

Darley, F. L., Aronson, A. E., & Brown, J. R. (1969b). Differential diagnostic patterns of dysarthria. *Journal of Speech and Hearing Research, 12*(2), 246–269. https://doi.org/10.1044/jshr.1202.246

De Bodt, M. S., Hernández-Díaz Huici, M. E., & Van De Heyning, P. H. (2002). Intelligibility as a linear combination of dimensions in dysarthric speech, *Journal of Communication Disorders, 35*(3), 283–292. https://doi.org/10.1016/S0021-9924(02)00065-5.

Diedrich, W. M. (1968). The mechanism of esophageal speech. *Annals of the New York Academy of Sciences, 155*(1), 303–317. https://doi.org/10.1111/j.1749-6632.1968.tb56776.x

Doyle, P. C. (Ed.). (2019). *Clinical care and rehabilitation in head and neck cancer.* Springer. https://doi.org/10.1007/978-3-030-04702-3

Doyle, P. C., Danhauer, J. L., & Reed, C. G. (1988). Listeners' perceptions of consonants produced by esophageal and tracheoesophageal talkers. *Journal of Speech and Hearing Disorders, 53*(4), 400–407. https://doi.org/10.1044/jshd.5304.400

Doyle, P. C., & Eadie, T. L. (2005). The perceptual nature of alaryngeal voice and speech. In P. C. Doyle & R. L. Keith (Eds.), *Contemporary considerations in the treatment and rehabilitation of head and neck cancer: Voice, speech, and swallowing* (pp. 113–140). Pro-Ed.

Doyle, P. C., & Finchem, E. A. (2019). Teaching esophageal speech: A process of collaborative instruction. In P. C. Doyle (Ed.), *Clinical care and rehabilitation in head and neck cancer* (pp. 145–161). Springer. https://doi.org/10.1007/978-3-030-04702-3

Duffy, J. R. (2019). *Motor speech disorders: Substrates, differential diagnosis, and management* (4th ed.). Elsevier Mosby.

Eadie T. L., & Doyle P. C. (2004). Auditory-perceptual scaling and quality of life in tracheoesophageal speakers. *The Laryngoscope, 114*(4), 753–759. https://doi.org/10.1097/00005537-200404000-00030

Eadie, T. L., Otero, D., Cox, S., Johnson, J., Baylor, C. R., Yorkston, K. M., & Doyle, P. C. (2016). The relationship between communicative participation and postlaryngectomy speech outcomes. *Head & Neck, 38*(S1), E1955–E1961. https://doi.org/10.1002/hed.24353

Evitts, P. M., & Gallop, R. (2011). Objective eye-gaze behavior during face-to-face communication with proficient alaryngeal speakers: A preliminary study. *International Journal of Language and Communication Disorders, 46*(5), 535–549. https://doi.org/10.1111/j.1460-6984.2011.00005.x

Evitts, P. M., Starmer, H., Teets, K., Montgomery, C., Calhoun, L., Schulze, A., . . . Adams, L. (2016). The impact of dysphonic voices on healthy listeners: Listener reaction times, speech intelligibility, and listener comprehension. *American Journal of Speech-Language Pathology, 25*(4), 561–575. https://doi.org/10.1044/2016_AJSLP-14-0183

Graville, D. J., Palmer, A. D., & Bolognone, R. K. (2019). Voice restoration with the tracheoesophageal voice prosthesis: The current state of the art. In P. C. Doyle (Ed.), *Clinical care and rehabilitation in head and neck cancer* (pp. 163–187). Springer. https://doi.org/10.1007/978-3-030-04702-3

Gress, C. D., & Singer, M. I. (2005). Tracheoesophageal voice restoration. In P. C. Doyle & R. L. Keith (Eds.), *Contemporary considerations in the treatment and rehabilitation of head and neck cancer: Voice, speech, and swallowing* (pp. 431–452). Pro-Ed.

Hillman, R. E., Walsh, M. J., Wolf, G. T., Fisher, S. G., & Hong, W. K. (1998). Functional outcomes following treatment for advanced laryngeal cancer: Part I—Voice preservation in advanced laryngeal cancer; Part II—Laryngectomy rehabilitation: The state of the art in the VA system. *Annals of Otology, Rhinology & Laryngology Supplement, 107*(5), 1–27.

Jacks, A. (2009). Acoustic correlates of prosodic abnormality in acquired apraxia of speech. *Perspectives in Neurophysiology and Neurogenic Speech and Language Disorders, 19*(3), 83–89. https://doi.org/10.1044/nnsld19.3.83

Lazarus, C. L. (2009). Effects of chemoradiotherapy on voice and swallowing. *Current Opinion in Otolaryngology & Head and Neck Surgery, 17*(3), 172–178. https://doi.org/10.1097/MOO.0b013e32832af12f

Max, L., Steurs, W., & de Bruyn, W. (1996). Vocal capacities in esophageal and tracheoesophageal speakers. *The Laryngoscope, 106*(1), 93–96. https://doi.org/10.1097/00005537-199601000-00018

Meltzner, G. S., & Hillman, R. E. (2005). Impact of aberrant acoustic properties on the perception of sound quality in electrolarynx speech. *Journal of Speech Language and Hearing Research, 48*(4), 766–779. https://doi.org/10.1044/1092-4388(2005/053)

Nagle, K. F. (2019). Elements of clinical training with the electrolarynx. In P. C. Doyle (Ed.), *Clinical care and rehabilitation in head and neck cancer* (pp. 129–143). Springer. https://doi.org/10.1007/978-3-030-04702-3

Perkell, J. S., Matthies, M. L., Svirsky, M. A., & Jordan, M. I. (1995). Goal-based speech motor control: A theoretical framework and some preliminary data. *Journal of Phonetics, 23*(1–2), 23–35. https://doi.org/10.1016/S0095-4470(95)80030-1

Perrier, P., & Fuchs, S. (2015). Motor equivalence in speech production. In M. A. Redford (Ed.), *The handbook of speech production* (pp. 223–247). Wiley Blackwell. https://doi.org/10.1002/9781118584156.ch11

Porcaro, C. K., Evitts, P. M., King, N., Hood, C., Campbell, E., White, L., & Veraguas, J. (2019). Effect of dysphonia and cognitive-perceptual listener strategies on speech intelligibility. *Journal of Voice, 34*(5), 806.e7–806.e18. https://doi.org/10.1016/j.jvoice.2019.03.013

Ramig, L. O. (1992). The role of phonation in speech intelligibility: A review and preliminary data from patients with Parkinson's disease. In R. D. Kent (Ed.), *Intelligibility in speech disorders: Theory, measurement and management* (pp. 119–155). John Benjamin.

Rong, P., Yunusova, Y., Wang, J., Zinman, L., Pattee, G. L., Berry, J. D., . . . Green, J. R. (2016). Predicting speech intelligibility decline in amyotrophic lateral sclerosis based on the deterioration of individual speech subsystems. *PLoS ONE, 11*(5), 1–19. https://doi.org/10.1371/journal.pone.0154971

Rosenbek, J. C. (1984). Treating the dysarthric talker. *Seminars in Speech and Language, 5*(4), 359–384. DOI: 10.1055/s-2008-1064294

Rothman, H. B. (1978). Analyzing artificial electronic larynx speech. In S. J. Salmon & L. P. Goldstein (Eds.), *The artificial larynx handbook* (pp. 87–111). Grune & Stratton.

Saikachi, Y., Stevens, K. N., & Hillman, R. E. (2009). Development and perceptual evaluation of amplitude-based F0 control in electrolarynx speech. *Journal of Speech, Language, and Hearing Research, 52*(5), 1360–1369. https://doi.org/10.1044/1092-4388(2009/08-0167)

Salmon, S. J. (2005). Commonalities among alaryngeal speech methods. In: P. C. Doyle & R. L. Keith (Eds.), *Contemporary considerations in the treatment and rehabilitation of head and neck cancer: Voice, speech, and swallowing* (pp. 59–74). Pro-Ed.

Sapienza, C. M., & Hoffman, B. (2022). *Voice disorders* (4th ed.). Plural Publishing.

Searl, J. (2017). Whispering by individuals using tracheoesophageal speech. *Journal of Voice, 32*(1), 127.e1–127.e13. https://doi.org/10.1016/j.jvoice.2017.04.007

Snidecor, J. C., & Curry, E. T. (1959). Temporal and pitch aspects of superior esophageal speech. *Annals of Otology, Rhinology, & Laryngology, 68*, 623–636. https://doi.org/10.1177/000348945906800302

Stachler, R. J., Francis, D. O., Schwartz, S. R., Damask, C. C., Digoy, G. P., Krouse, H. J., . . . Nnacheta, L. C. (2018). Clinical practice guideline: Hoarseness (Dysphonia) (Update) Executive summary. *Otolaryngology--Head and Neck Surgery. 158*(3), 409–426. https://doi.org/10.1177/0194599817751031

Trudeau, M. D., & Qi, Y. (1990). Acoustic characteristics of female tracheoesophageal speech. *Journal of Speech and Hearing Disorders, 55*(2), 244–250. https://doi.org/10.1044/jshd.5502.244

van As, C. J., Koopmans-van Beinum, F. J., Pols, L. C., & Hilgers, F. J. (2003). Perceptual evaluation of tracheoesophageal speech by naïve and experienced judges through the use of semantic differential scales. *Journal of Speech, Language, and Hearing Research, 46*(4), 947–959. https://doi.org/10.1044/1092-4388(2003/074)

van Sluis, K. E., van der Molen, L., van Son, R. J., Hilgers, F. J., Bhairosing, P. A., & van den Brekel, M. W. (2018). Objective and subjective voice outcomes after total laryngectomy: A systematic review. *European Archives of Oto-Rhino-Laryngology, 275*, 11–26. https://doi.org/10.1007/s00405-017-4790-6

Vos, T. G., Dillon, M. T., Buss, E., Rooth, M. A., Bucker, A. L., Dillon, S., . . . Dedmon, M. M.. (2021), Influence of protective face coverings on the speech recognition of cochlear implant patients. *The Laryngoscope, 131*, E2038–E2043. https://doi.org/10.1002/lary.29447

Vilaseca, I., Chen, A. Y., & Backscheider, A. G. (2006). Long-term quality of life after total laryngectomy. *Head Neck, 28*(4), 313–320. https://doi.org/10.1002/hed.20268

Weinberg, B. (1983). Voice and speech restoration following total laryngectomy. In W. H. Perkins (Ed.), *Voice disorders* (pp. 109–125). Thieme-Stratton.

Weismer, G. (Ed.). (2007). *Motor speech disorders*. Plural Publishing.

Williams, S. E., & Watson, J. B. (1987). Speaking proficiency variations according to method of alaryngeal voicing. *The Laryngoscope, 97*(6), 737–739. https://doi.org/10.1288/00005537-198706000-00018

World Health Organization (2001). *International Classification of Functioning, Disability, and Health.* https://www.who.int/standards/classifications/international-classification-of-functioning-disability-and-health

Yorkston, K. M., Beukelman, D. R., Strand, E. A., & Hakel, M. (2010). *Management of motor speech disorders in children and adults* (3rd ed.). Pro-Ed.

Ziegler, W., & von Cramon, D. (1986). Timing deficits in apraxia of speech. *European Archives of Psychiatry and Neurological Sciences, 236*, 44–49. https://doi.org/10.1007/BF00641058

Assessment of Speaker Structures and Functions: Subsystem Evaluation to Determine Contributions to Reduced Intelligibility

Key Points:

■ Asking case history questions based specifically on intelligibility can assist you in learning the impact of the client's reduced intelligibility to guide formation of a functional management plan.

■ Patient reported outcome measures provide practical information for pre-and post-treatment measures.

■ Using standardized recording protocols allows you to effectively compare pre-and post-treatment measures of intelligibility to determine effects of treatment.

■ Many measures, including standardized tests, rating scales, and applications can provide useful assessment information related to reduced intelligibility in our clients.

Understanding the factors that contribute to a speaker's reduced intelligibility is a critical component in forming a management plan. Speakers with reduced intelligibility will likely have a variety of issues related to the speech subsystems, so knowing what the client's strengths and areas for improvement are will help you decide what to target in treatment. This chapter covers evaluation of the speech subsystems to help you determine the impact that each might have on intelligibility. Beginning with a careful assessment of the speech subsystems will assist you in determining how to improve your client's intelligibility. To review, you might want to look back at Table 1–1 that describes the World Health Organization (2001) ICF classification system mentioned in Chapter 1. Using this system allows us to choose a starting place by examining the structures and functions of the speech subsystems. In completing an assessment, we want to learn as much as we can about the impairment that might be present in these functions and how it is impacting our client's ability to be understood. Assessment of subsystems is frequently associated with dysarthria but can also be used in the evaluation of clients with voice disorders as well as other disorders. As a clinician, you can use your judgment to determine which subsystems may require more in-depth assessment. This approach may not be as obviously helpful if you are dealing with reduced intelligibility in an alaryngeal speaker. Depending on the type of communication these speakers are using, there may be issues related primarily to the respiratory and articulatory subsystems. For patients dealing with H&N cancer, the consideration of subsystems will fall into very patient-specific considerations. In depth discussion and application of research related to subsystem influence on communication is available in *Clinical Care and Rehabilitation in Head and Neck Cancer*, edited by Doyle (2019). The assessment procedures in this chapter can help you collect baseline (pretreatment) information for clients, as well as an index of change that may occur over time or following treatment.

CASE HISTORY QUESTIONS

When you complete the case history with clients, questions focused on intelligibility may be helpful in determining a focus for management. Learning as much as you can about the client's reduced intelligibility and how it impacts their life will provide you valuable insight as you think about a management plan. Intelligibility-specific questions to be included are the following:

- Do people understand you better at different times of the day? For example, morning, mid-day, or evening?

- Do you communicate often for work? In person or by phone?

- Do you participate in social situations where you need to speak often?

- Who understands you the best?

- Who has the most difficulty understanding you?

- Are there specific situations where you feel you communicate better or worse?

- Are there specific sounds or words that you have more difficulty with?

- If people do not understand you, what strategies do you use to be understood?

Throughout the evaluation process, it's important to pay attention to the amount of stress, fatigue, and effort the client is experiencing. The case history and other parts of the evaluation will help to give you an idea of how severely the client's daily participation is being impacted, which can help you formulate a management plan.

STANDARDIZED TESTS AND RATING SCALES FOR SPEECH AND VOICE ASSESSMENT

Standardized tests and ratings scales may be useful to SLPs during assessment of speech and voice disorders. A standardized test or scale can provide a list of assessment tasks that may be helpful in examination of the subsystems. These measures may provide norms or ratings to help describe your client's level of impairment. However, there can be challenges to using these measures functionally. A main challenge for SLPs is that these tests and scales are not always available or affordable in clinical settings. We can use perceptual scales, but there can be subjectivity between two different raters or even between the same rater at different times. What one person hears as "mild" may be "moderate" to another. This subjectivity may carry into the words used to describe speech or voice characteristics. For example, one person might describe a voice as, "hoarse" and another person as, "harsh." To limit subjectivity, scales have been published to allow us to have more structure in our perceptual descriptions. Although this added structure can be helpful, it is important to remember that when using our "ears" for ratings, there will be subjectivity between raters. There are two types of scales commonly used to provide some level of objectivity to perceptual scales (Sapienza & Hoffman, 2022). We use an ordinal scale when numbers are linked with certain descriptors, for example, 0 =

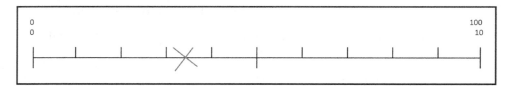

Figure 3–1. Example of a visual analog scale with clearly defined end points.

normal, 1 = mild, 2 = moderate, 3 = severe. We use a visual analog scale when a line with two endpoints is presented, and the rater draws a mark somewhere along that line to indicate the size or severity of the perceptual characteristic (Figure 3–1). Both types of scales have challenges and advantages but can help clinicians rate characteristics of clients in areas such as voice and speech.

Patient Reported Outcome Measures

Clinicians in various medical fields are increasingly using patient reported outcome (PRO) measures to include patient judgment in clinical decision-making. PRO measures involve gathering information about disabilities and their impact on participation and activities directly from the patient without interpretation from the clinician or family members (Snyder et al., 2013). The ICF framework discussed in Chapter 1 reminds us to consider multiple perspectives related to the impact of our client's disability and how important it is to learn about the experiences of the client. Donovan (2012) points out that several PRO measures allow insight into the societal participation of our clients, including the Communication Effectiveness Survey-Revised (CESR; Donovan, 2018) and the Communication Participation Index Bank (CPIB; Baylor et al., 2013). You will find the entire CESR in Appendix 3–1, and the short version of the CPIB in Appendix 3–2. SLPs who are interested in knowing more about the psychosocial impact of reduced intelligibility could use the Dysarthria Impact Profile (DIP; Walshe et al., 2009). We can gain insight into our client's physical perceptions and social experiences related to voice disorders, including alaryngeal speech, by using PRO measures designed for these types of clients. These include the Voice Related Quality of Life (V–RQOL; Hogikyan & Sethuraman, 1999) and the Voice Handicap Index (VHI; Jacobson et al., 1997). This perspective also aligns with our use of EBP to involve the client in goal setting and examination of progress. Yorkston et al. (2019) provides an excellent introduction of this topic and reminds us that large changes in test scores (or statistical significance in research) do not always align with meaningful change in the client's ability to communicate. Use of PRO measures can be an effective use of time to determine what change the client is experiencing related to treatment.

Published Dysarthria Measures

Speakers with dysarthria may exhibit difficulties in all subsystems, so you may want to include all areas in assessment. Table 3–1 provides a list of published assessment instruments SLPs can use with clients with dysarthria and a brief description of each. Many of these instruments focus on the evaluation of the subsystems and may include a measure of intelligibility. Table 3–2 contains PRO measures that have been formulated for use with clients with dysarthria.

Published Adult Apraxia of Speech Measures

Assessment of speakers with AAOS should focus on articulation and prosody, although other subsystems may affect those, so a broader approach may be best with these clients. There are few published assessments related to AAOS. Table 3–3 contains a brief list and description. Although not developed specifically for AAOS populations, there are general scales that may be helpful to gain insight into life impact of AAOS, including the CPIB (Baylor et al., 2013), which was developed to be used across different disorders. The Quality of Communication Life Scale (ASHA QCL) developed by Paul and colleagues (2004) for clients with aphasia and dysarthria could be used with clients diagnosed with AAOS.

Published Voice Disorders Measures

Speakers with voice disorders often demonstrate issues in the respiratory, phonatory, and resonatory subsystems. Prosody can be influenced by those as well. Instrumental measures, including acoustic, aerodynamic, and visualization, provide critical information related to diagnosis of voice disorders. However, clinicians may not have access to instrumentation or training to perform this portion of a voice evaluation. If instrumental measures are needed, we can refer clients to ENTs and/or SLPs who specialize in voice. Perceptual evaluation of voice frequently includes the use of scales to rate voice characteristics and patient perception of the voice disorder (PRO measure). Table 3–4 contains a list of published assessments and rating scales useful for clients with voice disorders, including H&N cancer. Patient reported outcome measures related to voice and H&N cancer are described in Table 3–5. Although some of the published measures developed for voice disorders may be useful for clients with H&N cancer, there are specific considerations for this population, including the location of tumor and type of treatment the client has undergone. Tables 3–4 and 3–5 contain information specific to an evaluation measure designed for and validated using participants with a diagnosis of H&N cancer.

Table 3–1. Instruments for Assessment of Dysarthria

Dysarthria Instrument	Authors, year published	Type of Measure	Description
* Frenchay Dysarthria Assessment (Second edition) FDA-2	Enderby & Palmer (2008)	Test battery completed by SLP	Examines: Reflexes, respiration, larynx, palate, tongue, and lips, as well as reflexes, rate, and intelligibility (word, sentence, and connected speech)
*Dysarthria Examination Battery (DEB)	Drummond (1993)	Test battery completed by SLP	Examines: Respiration, phonation, resonance, articulation, intelligibility (word and sentence), rate/prosody, and oral/tactile sensitivity
*Perceptual Dysarthria Evaluation (PDE)	Swigert (2010)	Test battery completed by SLP	Examines: Respiration, phonation, resonance, articulation, prosody. intelligibility, comprehensibility, and effectiveness (all rated for severity). Notes impact of environment on speech

Instrument	Source	Administration	Description
*Newcastle Dysarthria Assessment Tool (N-DAT)	Hackney & Vietch (2015)	Test battery completed by SLP	Examines: Respiration, phonation, resonance, prosody, articulation, and intelligibility (judged by SLP rating of client's connected speech sample). Findings interpreted using Dysarthria Differential Diagnosis Tool
Functional Communication Measures (FCM) Motor Speech Scale	American Speech-Language-Hearing Association (1995)	Rating scale completed by the SLP using a 7-point scale	Measures: Impact of dysarthria on communication while considering use of cueing methods and/or compensatory strategies. The FCMs are copyrighted for exclusive use so users must be enrolled in the data collection program through ASHA.
*Dysarthria Profile-Revised	Robertson & Thomson (1987)	Rating scale completed by SLP. Self-screening section completed by client and/or caregiver	Examines: Respiration, phonation, facial musculature, diadochokinesis, intelligibility, and rate/prosody. Self-screening: communication competence, eating/swallowing

Note: *Indicates instruments measuring intelligibility.

Table 3–2. Patient Related Outcome Measures of Dysarthria

Dysarthria Instrument	Authors, year published	Type of Measure	Description
*Dysarthria Profile-Revised	Robertson & Thomson (1987)	Rating scale completed by SLP Self-screening section completed by client and/or caregiver	Examines: Respiration, phonation, facial musculature, diadochokinesis, intelligibility, and rate/prosody Self-screening: communication competence, eating/swallowing
Communication Effectiveness Scale—Revised (CESR)	Donovan et al. (2007); Donovan (2018)	Rating scale consisting of 27 items completed by client using a 4-point scale	Measures: Effectiveness in various functional communication situations, including different conversational partners and different communication environments (telephone versus live conversations) (See Appendix 3–1)
Dysarthria Impact Profile	Walshe et al. (2009)	Rating scale consisting of 48 items completed by client	Measures: Effects of dysarthria on the client, acceptance of dysarthria by client, client perception of how others react to his/her speech, self-perceived impact of dysarthria on communication, and impact of dysarthria relative to other worries/concerns

Communication Participation Item Bank (CPIB)	Baylor et al. (2013)	Rating scale consisting of 46 items completed by client Short form includes 10 items	Provides: A single index of how client's communication interferes with participation in various situations. Developed to be a disorder-generic measure and examined initially with dysarthria and H&N cancer clients.
Living with Dysarthria	Hartelius et al. (2008)	Rating scale consisting of 50 items completed by client using a 5-point scale	Measures: Challenges related to dysarthria and cognitive-language issues, impact on speech by influences such as different listeners, emotional response, communicative environment/situation. Addresses how communication is impacted by the use of different strategies. Includes demographic and background information.
Quality of Communication Life Scale (ASHA QCL)	Paul et al. (2004)	Rating scale consisting of 19 total items, 8 directly related to communication completed by client using a 5-point scale	Measures: Quality of communication in social, work, education interaction and participation; as well as overall quality of life

Note: *Indicates both client measure and clinician measures (including intelligibility).

Table 3–3. Instruments for Assessment of Adult Onset Apraxia of Speech

Apraxia Instrument	Authors, year published	Type of Measure	Description
Apraxia Battery of Speech—2nd Edition (ABA-2)	Dabul (2000)	Test battery completed by SLP	Examines: Diadochokinetic rates, imitation of words of increasing length, latency and time of utterance naming pictured multisyllabic words, articulation during repetition of polysyllabic words, other speech behaviors, such as counting and reading
The Apraxia of Speech Rating Scale-3 (ASRS3)	Strand et al. (2014)	A 5-point rating scale is used to rate 16 items on presence/absence of AAOS characteristics, as well as prominence and severity.	Identifies: Differential diagnosis of AAOS and severity estimates by examining ■ Phonetic features Distortion, substitutions, additions and increasing length and complexity ■ Prosodic features Syllable segmentation Rate Lengthened segments ■ Other AMR/SMR disturbances Groping False starts and restarts Scores are provided by the SLP after listening to video and audio speech samples, including conversational speech, picture description, word and sentence repetition, and AMR/SMR tasks.

Table 3–4. Auditory-Perceptual Rating Measures of Voice Disorders and Head and Neck Cancer

Voice Instrument	Authors, year published	Type of Measure	Description
Consensus on Auditory Perceptual Evaluation of Voice (CAPE-V)	Kempster et al. (2009)	Visual Analog Scale of a 100-millimeter line. Standard recording methods are used to capture vowels, sentences, and conversational speech.	Describes: Auditory-perceptual characteristics of voice disorders, overall severity, roughness, breathiness, strain, pitch, and loudness. Ratings are also provided for consistent or intermittent occurrences of the characteristics.
GRBAS	Hirano (1981)	Rating scale consisting of 5 items completed by clinician using a 4-point scale	Measures severity in perceptual areas, including: (G) Grade on how disordered the voice sounds, (R) Roughness, (B) Breathiness, (A) Asthenia (weakness in vocal intensity), and (S) Strain
* London Speech Evaluation (LSE)	Dwivedi et al. (2012b)	Rating scale consisting of 5 parameters completed by clinician using a 4-point scale	Perceptual Speech Evaluation measuring intelligibility, articulation, speech rate, nasality, and asthenia of single words and connected speech.

Note: *Indicates measures validated on H&N cancer populations.

67

Table 3–5. Patient Reported Outcome Measures of Voice Disorders and Head and Neck Cancer

Voice Instrument	Authors, year published	Type of Measure	Description
Voice Handicap Index (VHI)	Jacobson et al. (1997)	Rating scale consisting of 30 items completed by client using a 5-point scale	Measures how a voice disorder affects quality of life, given three main areas: physical (how the voice sounds and feels), functional (impact on social and vocational), emotional (feeling about voice disorder)
Voice Handicap Index-10 (VHI-10)	Rosen et al. (2004)	Rating scale consisting of 10 items from the VHI completed by client	Same areas (physical, functional, and emotional) as VHI, found to found to be more powerful and less time-consuming than the original VHI
Voice Handicap Index-Partner (VHI-P)	Zraick et al. (2007)	Rating scale of 10 items derived from VHI completed by communication partner, independent of the client.	Same areas (physical, functional, and emotional) with ratings based on partner's perception.

Measure	Citation	Format	Description
Voice Symptom Scale (VoiSS)	Deary et al. (2003)	43 item questionnaire completed by client	Measures client reported voice severity in three main areas of impairment (voice disorder interference with life), emotional (feelings about voice disorder), and physical (discomfort, other symptoms)
Voice-Related Quality of Life (V-RQOL)	Hogikyan & Sethuraman (1999)	Rating scale consisting of 10 items completed by client using a 5-point scale	Measures severity and frequency of voice-related issues using two areas including a social-emotional domain and physical functioning domain
Voice Activity and Participation Profile (VAPP)	Ma & Yiu (2001)	28 item questionnaire completed by client	Measures client reported voice severity and level of impact on daily life in the following areas: job, daily communication, social communication and emotion.
* Speech Handicap Index (SHI)	Dwivedi et al. (2012a)	30 item questionnaire completed by client using a 5-point scale	Measures client reported speech impairments and related psycho-social impacts of speech impairment.

Note: *Indicates measures validated on H&N cancer populations.

FACTORS RELATED TO COLLECTING RECORDED SAMPLES

During an evaluation, SLPs should record a speech sample of their client. Your recording procedures can affect the accuracy of evaluation results. This section will cover aspects related to creating the best setup for recording clients in a clinical setting, given financial and technological challenges that are present in many facilities. Our goal is to create an optimal recording situation that we can replicate when we need to reevaluate. First of all, the client should sit comfortably in the quietest environment possible for recording. This may involve finding a different room or a time of day when there will be less background noise. If possible, do not have others in the room, but, if anyone else is present, they should be quiet. A tape or digital recorder or iPhone/iPad can be used, and your signal will be much better if you use a microphone. There are two types of microphones and it is helpful for you to know the difference, as your choice of which to use may be determined by the environment you will record in (Hunter et al., 2007). An omnidirectional microphone will pick up sounds from many directions, so it is not a good choice in a clinical recording environment with noise in the background. A unidirectional microphone is preferred in environments outside of those that are "sound treated" (e.g., sound booth) because it picks up sounds coming from a single direction. In a typical clinical setting, you can use a unidirectional microphone that is table mounted or head mounted. If you are going to have a microphone on your client's body, you have the choice of a lapel or head-mounted microphone. Some clients have extraneous head movements, such as someone with Parkinson's disease or Huntington's chorea. For these clients, you may want to use the lapel microphone to reduce noise in the recording caused by head movements.

In order to compare your recorded samples across different recording sessions, keep the microphone to mouth distance similar. You can measure the distance between your microphone and the client's mouth and note this so you can set it up the same distance for future recordings. Collecting a baseline sample with the microphone 24 inches from the client's mouth and a post treatment sample with the microphone two inches from the client's mouth might have you believing that the client's speech and voice have become clearer and louder. However, in reality, it could be that the recording procedures were not kept constant and that accounts for the differences you hear. If you keep the mouth to mic distance consistent, you will be more certain any changes you hear are not related to the recordings themselves. When reading this, you might think that a sound protected room isn't a "real life" environment where your client will communicate, as there is background noise that might be present in the client's normal communication environment. When you are working with your client, the background noise is something you will want to teach them about, and this topic is covered in depth in Chapter 8. However, when you are evaluating and want to compare recorded samples, you want a background that is similar in each recording. Background noise is difficult to control, so it is best to use the same protocol with a quiet environment and similar recording conditions each time you record.

Audio and visual recordings of clients can be very useful in assessment, but you need to consider client confidentiality issues related to these. The ASHA Code of Ethics (American Speech-Language-Hearing Association, 2016) contains several expectations that deal explicitly with patient confidentiality, including:

> Principle I, Rule O: Individuals shall protect the confidentiality and security of records of professional services provided, research and scholarly activities conducted, and products dispensed. Access to these records shall be allowed only when doing so is necessary to protect the welfare of the person or of the community, is legally authorized, or is otherwise required by law. (pp. 5–6)

> Principle I, Rule P: Individuals shall protect the confidentiality of any professional or personal information about persons served professionally or participants involved in research and scholarly activities and may disclose confidential information only when doing so is necessary to protect the welfare of the person or of the community, is legally authorized, or is otherwise required by law. (p. 6)

Using personal electronic devices, such as computers, phones, or flash drives to collect or store audio/visual recordings of clients is not conducive to keeping client data confidential. Your state board or employer may have policies or regulations about handling these types of records. There are privacy safeguards that can be used, such as password protection or client identifications that are anonymous. If you are allowed to record and use these safeguards, remember that the client's identity is available to anyone who can hear or see a recording of their physical appearance or voice.

Options for Recording Virtually

Increased use of telepractice has led to the creation of ways to collect speech and voice recordings in an online environment rather than live and in person. Many software platforms are available including WebEx and ZOOM, which are reported to be commonly used by SLPs for telepractice (Grillo, 2017). VoiceEvalU8 is an application (app) that works on smartphones and tablets through a server and web portal. This app allows SLPs to complete "mobile" voice evaluation, including a sustained vowel which is used to analyze fundamental frequency and other acoustic measures.

VoiceEvalU8 allows clinicians to gather perceptual measures using rating scales, such as the Voice Handicap Index (Jacobson, 1997) among others. Client measures of respiratory and phonatory measures can be collected as clients sustain /s/, /z/, and vowels. Elizabeth Grillo, who created the VoiceEvalU8, has completed research demonstrating its usefulness as a functional tool in effective recording and evaluation of clients with voice disorders (Grillo, 2017, 2019, 2021; Grillo & Wolfberg, 2020; Grillo et al., 2021. Schneider and colleagues (2021) provide useful suggestions for implementing voice recordings through telepractice. Technology is rapidly growing and providing SLPs with methods to allow clients to be seen in their home environments. Clinicians who plan to step into teletherapy as a new way to practice will find many resources in ASHA's evidence map related to telepractice (ASHA, n.d.).

Considerations When Recording With Face Masks

If masks are worn by both the clinician and the client, some adjustments in the recording protocol will be needed. We know that wearing a mask can reduce both the auditory/acoustic and visual information that would normally be available to listeners during face-to-face conversations (Corey et al., 2020; Vos et al., 2021). During an evaluation where masks are needed, following suggestions from Magee and colleagues (2020) can ensure that you capture the best audio and visual signal when you are recording your client. While both of you are masked, assist the client in getting the microphone set up and in place. Be sure the microphone is not touching the client's face if you are using a head–mounted device. Step away from the client for social distancing and ask the client to carefully remove their mask during recording.

AUDITORY–PERCEPTUAL EVALUATION

As our ultimate goal is for a listener's ears to understand our clients, you may want to use informal auditory-perceptual measures to evaluate the subsystems. SLPs could include these measures to supplement information obtained from more formal measures. A description of the auditory-perceptual characteristics and severity of impairment of the subsystems will be a useful target for an assessment of clients with reduced intelligibility. The following section provides descriptions of auditory-perceptual measures that can be completed for each of the subsystems of speech without using a published test or scale. This type of evaluation allows clinicians to complete real-world, functional measures of their client's speech and voice. Clinicians can use their knowledge of disorders to determine which subsystems may require more focus. Duffy (2019) suggests completing a thorough case history and obtaining recorded samples of various speech tasks, including vowel prolongation, alternating motion rates (AMRs), and connected speech through reading or conversation.

Evaluation of Respiration

It is critical for SLPs to have a good understanding of the client's ability to utilize their respiratory system to support speech because this system provides the driving force behind speech production. SLPs can use our ears and eyes to make careful observations and measures of how efficiently clients use respiration for speech.

Posture and Body Movement Observation

Observe the patient's posture while standing and sitting. Pay attention to any factors that may keep them from sitting in an upright position. Look for signs of slumping to one side or being slouched down while seated. Lack of an upright posture can restrict the movements that are needed to support speech. Watch for signs of abnormal or inefficient breathing patterns during conversation. Normal speech breathing occurs with movements from both the abdomen and rib cage wall, although individuals vary how much each of these contributes (Hixon & Hoit, 2005). Clavicular breathing occurs when there is elevation of the shoulders during inhalation, and this is not considered to be an efficient respiratory pattern. If you see this pattern, make note of the circumstance and probe to see if the client can change the movements when directed to limit shoulder movements.

Duration Measures

Many resources, including Duffy's 2019 textbook on motor speech disorders, suggest using durational or timed measures to examine the respiratory-phonatory systems for speech. Use of maximum phonation duration (MPD), also called maximum phonation time (MPT), gives us an idea of the maximum amount of air a client can generate for phonation. To measure MPD, ask the client to "take a deep breath and say 'ah' for as long as you can until you are completely out of air." While the client is completing this task, you can use a stopwatch to time how many seconds they prolong the vowel. Kent and colleagues (1987) summarized data from studies of MPD of young and elderly (over age 65) and reported the following range of scores: young males, 22.6 to 34.6 seconds; young females, 15.2 to 26.5; elderly males, 13.0 to 18.1 seconds; and elderly females, 10.0 to 15.4 seconds. These authors noted that this measure is influenced by many factors, including how many times the client has practiced the task, whether the clinician has modeled the task, if the clinician is providing encouragement to the client during the task (example, "keep going, you can say it longer"), and the client's level of motivation. As there are many factors that influence MPD, if you are using it as an evaluation measure, consider giving one example after explaining the task to guide the client. MPD varies quite a lot between clients and under different conditions, and Duffy (2019) suggests that durations that are longer than nine seconds can be considered normal.

Breath Group Measures

We define a breath group as the number of syllables (or words) that a person can produce on one breath. SLPs can measure breath groups by having the client read or speak conversationally and then counting the number of syllables/words produced on one breath. The larger the number, the more air the client has ready and under control for speech (Hixon & Hoit, 2005). However, there is large variability between speakers, related to age, gender, and many other factors, including loudness, rate, and pauses in speech (Hoit & Hixon, 1987; Huber & Darling-White, 2017). For a general measure, Swigert (2010) suggests that speakers who produce less than 12 to 20 syllables per breath might experience laryngeal valving or velopharyngeal closure issues. For our purposes related to intelligibility, having a "norm" for syllables per breath isn't necessary. We are taking a measure of breath groups to ensure that clients can use respiratory support to allow others to understand their speech. For this reason, the actual number of syllables per breath is helpful, but what we really need to consider is whether the breath support is contributing to reduced intelligibility. For example, if the client is less intelligible when running out of air at the end of phrases or sentences, this should be noted. This person may need to take more breaths, which actually translates to a smaller number of breath groups, but may increase intelligibility.

Conversational and Reading Measures Related to Respiration

By using conversational or reading samples, SLPs can assess several measures related to respiration. During the evaluation, it is important to pay attention to the loudness level of the client in several communication settings to determine if they can vary their loudness appropriately. One cause of decreased loudness is poor respiratory support, as loudness of speech is an indicator of the strength and force of the respiratory system (Hixon & Hoit, 2005). In assessing loudness, consider whether the client's voice is too loud or too quiet for the communication environment. A speaker should be loud enough to be heard over background noise, but not so loud that listeners feel discomfort or are distracted (Awan, 2001). A sound pressure level (SPL) meter can be purchased inexpensively to provide measures of the client's loudness. You are measuring decibels of sound pressure level (dB SPL) which is what we perceive as loudness. These devices are priced from $20.00 to much higher if you search the Internet. There are apps available that will give measures of dB SPL. If you are using one of these devices, ensure that you place it at a similar distance from the client across recordings to ensure comparable measures. Typical conversational speech ranges from 65 to 80 dB SPL (Baken, 1996). Boone and colleagues (2019) remind us that older adults may have slightly less intense conversational speech levels. Calibration is important if you are using a SPL meter, but it is beyond the scope of this book. You can find helpful information in tutorials by Maryn and Zarowski (2015) and Švec and Granqvist (2018).

If the client is not using an appropriate loudness level, determine if the client can vary by it asking them to repeat words or phrases with the same loudness you use. You can ask the client to produce "ah" starting in a quiet voice and moving toward a loud voice. During the entire session, and hopefully across different environments, you can listen to determine if the client is able to vary loudness level appropriately.

There are other perceptual observations you can make either during the evaluation or when listening to recorded speech samples. Stridor or audible inspiration (or inhalation) occurs when there is a discoordination between the respiratory and phonatory systems. Stridor may be heard if there is an obstruction or constriction in the airway, such as stenosis (i.e., narrowing) of the trachea. When you hear stridor, it sounds like phonation during inhalation/inspiration and it can be very distracting to listeners. If a client has decreased breath support, you may hear short phrases with breaths in between. Or, the speech may trail off at the ends of sentences, and listeners might not understand because of the low loudness level near the end.

Evaluation of Phonation

Although some measures discussed in the evaluation of respiration section will overlap or interact with measures of phonation, there are many aspects that should be considered individually. In our field, we consider three important aspects of phonation, including loudness, pitch, and quality. Perceptual observation and measures of these areas can be completed if you listen to your client's voice during the assessment and/or record them on various tasks, including vowel prolongation and conversational speech. If you have access to instrumentation related to voice assessment, Patel and colleagues (2018) is an excellent resource to help you develop a protocol for assessment of vocal function.

Measures of Loudness

Both the phonatory and respiratory systems play a role in vocal intensity or loudness. According to Stemple et al. (2014), vocal intensity is influenced by the lateral movements (opening) of the vocal folds and how quickly they return to the closed position. These movements result from the amount and pressure of subglottal air (respiratory pressure that builds up under the closed vocal folds). In observing our client's loudness level and ability to vary loudness, we are gathering information regarding both the respiratory and phonatory systems. Asking clients to vary loudness while changing respiration, such as taking a deeper breath to get louder, may give some insight into management, but it is likely that you will not really separate these two subsystems when you assess or treat loudness issues.

Measures of Pitch

During conversational speech, SLPs should listen for a client's pitch to determine if it seems appropriate for the client's body size, gender, and other factors. Frequency is determined by how fast our vocal folds are vibrating, in fact fundamental frequency is how many times the vocal folds open and close per second. We measure frequency in hertz (Hz). Pitch is the term we use to describe what we perceive for frequency. A larger or taller person might have vocal folds with more mass and length, so we would expect that person to have a fairly low pitch, as those vocal folds cannot vibrate as quickly as compared to those of a smaller individual. This explains why men generally have lower pitch than women, and children have the highest pitch of all three groups. Vocal folds that have swelling or growths will also not vibrate as quickly as normal due to the extra mass, so individuals with dysphonia often demonstrate pitches that are lower than the person's normal level. We also want to listen for variation in pitch that we commonly use to show inflection. If the person is not using variation of pitch, we would report this as monopitch or monotone.

If you want to add some simple acoustic measures, you can find apps that measure pitch, costing between $1.00 to $5.00. You can also download a free software program called Praat (Boersma & Weenink, 2021) that allows you to measure frequency (pitch), intensity (loudness) and other voice parameters. You can download Praat at http://www.praat.org. Praat is a somewhat user-friendly program. You may need assistance in using it and you will find several helpful tutorials if you search online for instructions. If you use an app to measure your client's fundamental frequency, it's helpful to have an idea of what is considered "normal." The average speaking fundamental frequency for adult males ranges from 89.0 to 175.0 Hz, and for adult females from 164.5 to 260.0 Hz (Boone et al., 2019).

Patients who have disordered phonation may, at times, demonstrate diplophonia, which means "double voice" (Colton et al., 2011). This occurs when the vocal folds are not vibrating in the same manner for various reasons and can actually sound like two different pitches at the same time. SLPs should also listen for a vocal tremor, which may be much more noticeable during a vowel prolongation than when the client is speaking words and sentences. During connected speech, the tremor may not be as easily heard because the client is producing voiced and voiceless sounds throughout. During a vowel prolongation, the tremor is often more easily noticed when there are no voiceless sounds.

Measures of Quality

Measuring the quality of someone's voice can present several challenges. One is that in real-world, clinical situations, SLPs do not always have access to instrumentation, so they may rely on the use of rating scales and similar systems of describing voice quality. Another challenge is that in using these scales and descriptors, we must agree on common language to describe what we hear in a person's voice. People use terms like "breathy" and "hoarse" to describe voices, but not everyone uses them in the same way. Voice rating scales, such as those described in Table 3–4, allow SLPs to have lists of voice qualities to listen for, and some also provide numerical ratings linked to severity of these qualities. Common descriptors include breathy, harsh, strained-strangled, hoarse, glottal fry, hard glottal attacks, and aphonia (lack of phonation). A committee of members of ASHA's Special Interest Group 3, Voice and Voice Disorders developed the Consensus Auditory-Perceptual Evaluation of Voice (CAPE–V; Kempster et al., 2009). Lack of consensus in voice descriptors led to the creation of the CAPE–V, and the committee who created it consisted of specialists and researchers in voice. Members of ASHA can download the CAPE–V form and a description of the vocal attributes and policies for using the scale in a standardized format. None of the voice scales listed in this chapter was designed to be the only measure of voice quality, but they can complement other aspects of a voice examination.

Evaluation of Resonance

In order to describe or measure resonance, we should first define the term in relation to our clients with voice or speech disorders. Kummer (2006) describes resonance as "the quality of the voice that is determined by the balance of sound vibration in the oral, nasal, and pharyngeal cavities during speech." When we listen to a conversational speech sample, we want to focus on where the signal is resonating in the speaker's vocal tract. One of the more obvious descriptor words we use is hypernasality, which is used to describe nasal resonance in excess or on sounds that should not be nasalized. We sometimes hear nasal emissions of air as breath moves through the nasal passages and out the nose during speech. A nasal emission can be heard as a puff of air from the nose in addition to the oral signal. Nasal emission can be heard on plosives, fricatives, and affricates because those sounds involve building up oral pressure, which can escape through the nasal cavity. We use the term hyponasal or denasal to describe how a voice sounds when the nasal consonants (/m/, /n/, /ŋ/) do not have nasalization. Oral cul-de-sac resonance occurs when there is a posterior positioning of the tongue, resulting in the sound being focused in the oral pharyngeal area. To listen for all the descriptors of resonance, you should be sure that the client produces consonants that are nasal/oral and pressure consonants. An example of a sentence with many nasal sounds is "Mary is making new muffins." The sentence, "Be good to other people." contains no nasal sounds. If you feel you need some guidance on assessment of a client's resonance, check out the scales and instruments listed in Tables 3–1 and 3–4. Many contain items related to ratings of resonance.

One way to determine if nasality is impacting intelligibility is to occlude the client's nostrils during speech and listen to them produce vowels or connected speech. If you understand more or the voice sounds improved with the nostrils occluded, consider that nasality is impacting intelligibility (Swigert, 2010). SLPs can place a mirror under the client's nose while they produce non-nasalized pressure consonants, such as the word "puppy." The SLP should note that some fogging may occur even with normal resonance, but we may notice excessive amounts with this method, which correlates with both auditory-perceptual ratings of nasality and with instrumental measures using nasometry (Chow et al., 2015).

Evaluation of Articulation

Speech-Like Movements and Rates

For many clients with reduced intelligibility, we will want to assess articulation skills in several ways to provide useful clinical information that will lead to optimal management. Use of AMRs, SMRs or diadochokinetic rates allows us to observe the movements of the jaw, lip, and tongue in speech-like tasks. Duffy (2019) notes they also provide us with information on precision of articulation, respiratory and phonatory support for speech, and the client's ability to generate intraoral pressure for plosive sounds. In assessing AMRs, we should ask the client to repeatedly produce the following syllables, "puh," "tuh," and "kuh." You should instruct the client to take a deep breath and produce as many of each syllable as possible. Provide a model so the client will have a good understanding of the task. You can determine the number of repetitions per second by using a stopwatch.

Kent et al. (1987) summarized AMR norms for young and elderly adults as "puh" 5.0 to 7.1 repetitions per second; "tuh" 4.8 to 7.1 repetitions per second; 'kuh" 4.4 to 6.4 repetitions per second.

Sequential motion rates (SMRs) provide information on the client's ability to move the articulators quickly and sequentially in different positions. In this task, we ask the client to take a deep breath and repeat "puh-tuh-kuh puh-tuh-kuh" until you ask them to stop. A model from the clinician will help the client understand the task. Norms for young and elderly adults range from 3.6 to 7.5 repetitions per second (Kent et al., 1987). SMR measures can be especially helpful with patients who may have AAOS, as planning/programming is required in this task. You should pay attention to a large performance difference between AMRs and SMRs as more difficulty with SMRs might suggest AAOS. SLPs should observe both speed and regularity of rhythm of AMRs and SMRs as both provide information related to the client's speech-like movements.

Speech Sound Inventory

Depending on the type of disorder and the client, it may be helpful to have an inventory of speech sound errors. The Fisher-Logemann Test of Articulation (FLTA) Competence (Fisher & Logemann, 1971) can provide an extensive account of the client's ability to produce consonants and vowels in initial, medial, and final positions. If a client has inconsistent error or distortions, the FLTA or a similar test may not be helpful, and it can be time consuming to administer. However, it may provide SLPs with useful phonetic information in clients where articulatory patterns would be targets of management, such as oral cancer (Constantinescu & Rieger, 2019). Kent and colleagues (1989) designed two single word intelligibility tests designed with sets of minimal phonetic contrasts that can help clinicians determine which sounds are in error and impacting intelligibility.

Connected Speech Sample

A connected speech sample can help you assess other areas related to articulation, as well as the other subsystems. You will elicit some connected speech during the case history and throughout the evaluation. Plan some open-ended questions that will allow you to hear connected speech samples. You can ask about hobbies, family, travel, or other interest areas. Reading passages can be used to collect samples of speech as well, although some clients may have difficulty with that task. Recording the sample will allow you to go back and review at a later time. Listen for articulation errors, including imprecise consonants, irregular breakdowns, and vowel distortions. You may also get an idea of specific sounds that might be problematic for the client, and you can target those with lists of words or sentences containing those sounds. Are there consistent errors that you observe? Words and sentences with increasing length and complexity will be useful in clients where you suspect AAOS may be present. It may be useful to attempt some stimulability testing to determine if the client can produce difficult sounds correctly, given your model.

Evaluation of Prosody

Prosody has been found to be an important factor contributing to intelligibility and communicative effectiveness in adults with dysarthria, making it a critical part of assessment (Patel, 2002; Patel & Campellone, 2009). When determining if a client has appropriate prosody in their speech, you will examine the subsystems of respiration, phonation, and articulation. Listening to a sample of connected speech is one of the best ways for us to assess prosody. There are four parameters to include in an assessment of prosody (Swigert, 2010), including stress, intonation, rate, and rhythm. To examine stress, we listen for whether the client can use pitch, loudness, and/or duration to emphasize syllables or words. For example, if you say to the client, "It's nice to meet you, Mr. Jones" but his last name is Smith, you might expect he will correct you by saying, "My name is Smith" with emphasis on his name. We expect speakers to use pitch inflections in conversation that reflect your client's ability to use intonation. We might use rising inflection at the end of a question, which helps listeners know we are asking a question. Determining if your client uses intonation appropriately can be accomplished by listening for changes in pitch or a limitation in this (monotone). A perceptual judgment of rate is made when you determine if your client's speech sounds abnormally fast or slow. To assess rhythm, listen to see if speech is smooth and connected versus choppy (Swigert, 2010). Determining the speaker's ability to compensate for prosodic errors will be helpful in forming a plan for management (Patel, 2011).

SUMMARY

If we are using assessment methods to document pre-treatment (baseline) to compare with post-treatment measures, it is important to be aware of factors, such as recording methods that may need to be kept constant each time we collect data. To fully understand what is contributing to our client's reduced intelligibility, we need a thorough assessment of all subsystems involved. Deciding which subsystems to evaluate and how to do so is a task that is specific for each client. Clinicians can use standardized assessments and/or less formal measures to gain understanding of what to target in management. The use of PRO measures allows us to have greater knowledge of the impact of the reduced intelligibility on the client's participation level and activities that involve communication.

Case Study

Dysarthria Case: Jack's SLP, Christy, administered the Perceptual Dysarthria Examination (PDE; Swigert, 2010) because it allowed for a thorough evaluation of the subsystems involved in his case, including severity level ratings. Each subsystem has a section where the SLP selects physiologic characteristics that are observed in the client. The results from the PDE administered to Jack included the following:

Respiration:

- ■ PDE Rating—moderate
  - ▫ Short phrases secondary to reduced breath support
  - ▫ Reduced loudness

Phonation:

- ■ PDE Rating—mild
  - ▫ Pitch—within normal limits
  - ▫ Loudness—reduced loudness
  - ▫ Quality—breathy

Resonation:

- ■ PDE Rating—moderate
  - ▫ Hypernasality

Articulation:

- ■ PDE Rating—mild
  - ▫ Imprecise consonants

Prosody:

- ■ PDE Rating—mild
  - ▫ Excess and equal stress
  - ▫ Flat intonation

The case history section of the PDE provided Christy with useful information about Jack's challenges with communication. He reported that his speech was worse when he was stressed or tired and usually worse at the end of the day. He experienced the most difficulties talking with people who did not know him well and with most people (other than his immediate family) on the phone. He reported it bothered him significantly when people did not understand him and either asked him to repeat or just pretended to understand. He frequently avoided social situations that he would have liked to attend and evaded interacting in class. In responding to what was helpful, he said slowing down seemed to help listeners understand him. He reported that he has, at times, resorted to writing down words not understood. Although he stated that written information helped his listeners understand him, he did not like to do this. Table 3–6 shows how ICF can be applied to assessment of Jack's impairments and limitations.

Table 3–6. ICF Application for Jack's Case

Health Condition	Activity and Participation Limitations
■ Traumatic Brain Injury	■ Reduced intelligibility
Impairments	Contextual Factors
■ Muscle Functions	■ Technology capable
■ Speech Functions	■ Strong family support

Source: World Health Organization (2001).

Case Study

Voice Disorders Case: Thomas, the SLP, received a referral from Beth's ENT for her to participate in voice therapy. After an initial phone call, Thomas and Beth mutually decided that telepractice was the only option for her to participate in treatment. Thomas was both an experienced voice specialist and telepractitioner. The skills he utilized often during teletherapy included using the white board, screen sharing, recording, and editing as needed to share with clients. The practice where Thomas worked had access to a high-definition video connection with a secure, encrypted platform. Beth's daughter worked in information technology and agreed to assist with her mother's treatment by serving as an eHelper to ensure the proper set up and use of technology during the sessions.

A face-to-face voice evaluation was not possible, so Thomas arranged a three–person telepractice consultation between himself, Beth, and her ENT. Following a clear discussion of the ENT report and Beth's goals, Thomas felt comfortable providing teletherapy sessions to address her voice disorder, focusing on allowing her to return to her normal social and family life. Before beginning sessions, Thomas, Beth, and her daughter communicated by phone to adjust the settings on her computer and in the video platform to allow for her voice to be heard most effectively over background noises. Thomas recommended a sound pressure level (SPL), which Beth purchased to measure SPL targets during treatment sessions.

The ENT evaluation report sent to Thomas indicated moderate bowing of the vocal folds and mild decrease in the mucosal wave movement. Thick mucus was seen in the hypopharynx, which may have indicated inadequate hydration. Thomas completed evaluation measures with Beth using a secure, encrypted system and carefully noting the settings to replicate when he completed further testing. Thomas recorded Beth reading content from the Consensus Auditory–Perceptual Evaluation of Voice (CAPE–V; Kempster et al., 2009). He chose this rating scale because each of the parameters on the CAPE–V can be judged using audiovisual modalities utilized during telepractice (Myers et al., 2022). He rated the sample, and an overall severity score of 27/100 was obtained indicating mild-to-moderate impairment of voice. Ratings of perceptual features were as expected for age-related voice changes, including moderate roughness, mild-moderate strain and mild-moderate decreased loudness. Thomas asked Beth to complete the Voice Handicap Index (VHI; Jacobson et al., 1997) and her scores corresponded with mild severity in functional and emotional sections, moderate in the physical section, and mild-moderate self-perceived voice handicap overall. Beth stated that her frustration level was increasing as she had to "give up" more activities due to not being understood. Following successful trial therapy to stimulate louder voice without strain, Thomas recommended Beth begin voice teletherapy twice a week for age-related voice changes.

REFERENCES

American Speech-Language-Hearing Association. (n.d.). Telepractice. *ASHA's Evidence Maps.* https://www2.asha.org/EvidenceMapLanding.aspx?id=858 9944872&recentarticles=false&year=undefined&tab=all

American Speech-Language-Hearing Association. (1995). *ASHA National Outcomes Measurement System (NOMS) Functional Communication Measures (FCMs) Motor Speech Scale.* https://coe.uoregon.edu/cds/files/2013/12 /ASHA–NOMS.pdf

American Speech-Language-Hearing Association. (2016). *Code of Ethics* [Ethics]. Available from http://www.asha.org/policy

Awan, S. N. (2001). *The voice diagnostic protocol: A practical guide to the diagnosis of voice disorders.* Aspen.

Baken, R. J. (1996). *Clinical measurement of speech and voice.* College Hill Press.

Baylor, C., Yorkston, K., Eadie, T., Kim, J., Chung, H., & Amtmann, D. (2013). The Communicative Participation Item Bank (CPIB): Item bank calibration and development of a disorder-generic short form. *Journal of Speech, Language, and Hearing Research, 56*(4), 1190–1208. https://doi .org/10.1044/1092–4388(2012/12–0140)

Boersma, P., & Weenink, D. (2021). *Praat: Doing phonetics by computer* [Computer program]. Version 6.1.50. http://www.praat.org

Boone, D. R., McFarlane, S. C., Von Berg, S. L., & Zraick, R. I. (2019). *The voice and voice therapy* (10th ed.). Pearson.

Chow, W., Brandt, M. G., Dworschak-Stokan, A., Doyle, P. C., Matic, D., & Husein, M. (2015). Validation of the mirror-fogging test as a screening tool for velopharyngeal insufficiency. *The Open Otorhinolaryngology Journal, 8*, 15–21.

Colton, R. H., Casper, J. K., & Leonard, R. (2011). *Understanding voice problems: A physiological perspective for diagnosis and treatment* (4th ed.). Lippincott Williams & Wilkins.

Constantinescu, G., & Rieger, J. M. (2019). Speech deficits associated with oral and oropharyngeal carcinomas. In P. C. Doyle (Ed.), *Clinical care and rehabilitation in head and neck cancer.* (pp. 265–279). Springer. https://doi.org/10.1007/978–3–030–04702–3_16

Corey, R. M., Jones, U., & Singer, A. C. (2020). Acoustic effects of medical, cloth, and transparent face masks on speech signals. *The Journal of the Acoustical Society of America, 148*(4), 2371–2375. https://doi.org/10.1121/10.0002279

Dabul, B. L. (2000). *Apraxia Battery for Adults–Second Edition (ABA–2): Manual.* Pro–Ed.

Deary, I. J., Wilson, J. A., Carding, P. N., & MacKenzie, K. (2003). VoiSS: A patient–derived voice symptom scale. *Journal of Psychosomatic Research, 54*(5), 483–489. https://doi.org/10.1016/S0022–3999(02)00469–5

Donovan, N. J. (2012). Patient–reported outcomes for acquired dysarthria. *Perspectives on Neurophysiology and Neurogenic Speech and Language Disorders, 22*(4), 152–159. https://doi.org/10.1044/nnsld22.4.152

Donovan, N. J. (2018). Examining the item–level psychometrics properties of the Communication Effectiveness Survey–Revised for people with Parkinson's disease and dysarthria. *Clinical Archives of Communication Disorders, 3*(1), 42–51. http://dx.doi.org/10.21849/cacd.2018.00269

Donovan, N. J., Velozo, C. A., & Rosenbek, J. C. (2007). The Communicative Effectiveness Survey: Investigating its item–level psychometric properties. *Journal of Medical Speech–Language Pathology, 15*(4), 433–447.

Doyle, P. C. (Ed.). (2019). *Clinical care and rehabilitation in head and neck cancer.* Springer. https://doi.org/10.1007/978–3–030–04702–3

Drummond, S. S. (1993). *Dysarthria examination battery (DEB): Manual.* Communication Skill Builders.

Duffy, J. R. (2019). *Motor speech disorders: Substrates, differential diagnosis, and management* (4th ed.). Elsevier.

Dwivedi, R. C., St. Rose, S., Chisholm, E. J., Bisase, B., Amen, F., Nutting, C. M., . . . Kazi, R. (2012a). Evaluation of speech outcomes using English version of the Speech Handicap Index in a cohort of head and neck cancer patients. *Oral Oncology, 48*(6), 547–553. https://doi.org/10.1016/j.oraloncology.2012.01.001

Dwivedi, R. C., St. Rose, S., Chisholm, E. J., Kerawala, C. J., Clarke, P. M., Nutting, C. M., . . . Kazi, R. (2012b). Development and validation of first-ever speech-specific perceptual speech evaluation tool for patients with head and neck cancer: The London Speech Evaluation (LSE) scale. *Head & Neck, 34*(1), 94–103. https://doi.org/10.1002/hed.21683

Enderby, P., & Palmer, R. (2008). *Frenchay Dysarthria Assessment–Second Edition (FDA–2): Manual.* Pro–Ed.

Fisher, H. B., & Logemann, J. A. (1971). *The Fisher-Logemann Test of Articulation Competence (FLTA): Manual.* Pro–Ed.

Grillo, E. U. (2017). Results of a survey offering clinical insights into speech-language pathology telepractice methods. *International Journal of Telerehabilitation, 9*(2), 25–30. https://doi. org/10.5195/ijt.2017.6230

Grillo, E.U. (2019). Building a successful voice telepractice program. *Perspectives of the ASHA Special Interest Groups (SIG 3), 4*(1), 100–110. https://www.ncbi.nlm.nih.gov/pmc/articles/PMC6754185//

Grillo, E.U. (2021). Functional voice assessment and therapy methods supported by telepractice, VoiceEvalU8, and Estill Voice Training. *Seminars in Speech and Language, 42*(1), 41–53. https://www.ncbi.nlm.nih.gov/pmc/articles/PMC8417890//

Grillo, E. U., & Wolfberg, J. (2020). An assessment of different Praat versions for acoustic measures analyzed automatically by VoiceEvalU8 and manually by two raters. *Journal of Voice* [Advance online publication]. https://doi.org/10.1016/j.jvoice.2020.12.003

Grillo, E.U., Corej, B., & Wolfberg, J. (2021). Normative values of client-reported outcome measures and self-ratings of six voice parameters via the VoiceEvalU8 app. *Journal of Voice*. Advance online publication. https://doi.org/10.1016/j.jvoice.2021.10.026

Hackney, W., & Vietch, K. (2015*). Newcastle Dysarthria Assessment Tool (N–DAT)*. NSW Adult Speech Pathology Acquired Communication Impairment EBP Group. https://nswspeechpathologyebp.files.wordpress.com/2015/10/newcastle–ebp–dysarthria–assessment–tool–n–dat–dec–2015.pdf

Hartelius, L., Elmberg, M., Holm, R., Lövberg, A. S., & Nikolaidis, S. (2008). Living with dysarthria: Evaluation of a self–report questionnaire. *Folia Phoniatrica et Logopaedica, 60*(1), 11–19. https://doi.org/10.1159/000111799

Hirano, M. (1981). *Clinical examination of voice.* Springer.

Hixon, T. J., & Hoit, J. D. (2005). *Evaluation and management of speech breathing disorders: Principles and methods.* Redington Brown.

Hogikyan, N. D., & Sethuraman, G. (1999). Validation of an instrument to measure voice-related quality of life (V–RQOL). *Journal of Voice, 13*(4), 557–569. https://doi.org/10.1016/S0892–1997(99)80010–1

Hoit, J. D., & Hixon, T. J. (1987). Age and speech breathing. *Journal of Speech, Language, and Hearing Research, 30*(3), 351–366. https://doi.org/10.1044/jshr.3003.351

Huber, J. E., & Darling-White, M. (2017). Longitudinal changes in speech breathing in older adults with and without Parkinson's disease. *Seminars in Speech and Language, 38*(3), 200–209. https://doi.org/10.1055/s–0037–1602839

Hunter, E. J., Spielman, J., Starr, A., & Popolo, P. (2007). Acoustic voice recording, "I am seeking recommendations for voice recording hardware...". *Perspectives on Voice and Voice Disorders, 17*(3), 7–14. https://doi.org/10.1044/vvd17.3.7

Jacobson, B. H., Johnson, A., Grywalski, C., Silbergleit, A., Jacobson, G., Benninger, M. S., & Newman, C. W. (1997). The Voice Handicap Index (VHI): Development and validation. *American Journal of Speech–Language Pathology, 6*(3), 66–70. https://doi.org/10.1044/1058–0360.0603.66

Kempster, G. B., Gerratt, B. R., Verdolini Abbott, K., Barkmeier-Kraemer, J., & Hillman, R. E. (2009). Consensus Auditory-Perceptual Evaluation of Voice: Development of a standardized clinical protocol. *American Journal of Speech–Language Pathology, 18*(2), 124–132. https://doi.org/10.1044/1058–0360(2008/08–0017)

Kent, R. D., Kent, J. F., & Rosenbek, J. C. (1987). Maximum performance tests of speech production. *Journal of Speech and Hearing Disorders, 52*(4), 367–387.

Kent, R. D., Weismer, G., Kent, J. F., & Rosenbek, J. C. (1989). Toward phonetic intelligibility testing in dysarthria. *Journal of Speech and Hearing Disorders, 54*(4), 482–499. https://doi.org/10.1044/jshd.5404.482

Kummer, A. W. (2006). Resonance disorders and nasal emissions: Evaluation and treatment using "low tech" and "no tech" procedures. *The ASHA Leader, 11*(2). https://doi.org/10.1044/leader.FTR1.11022006.4

Ma, E. P. M., & Yiu, E. M. L. (2001). Voice activity and participation profile: Assessing the impact of voice disorders on daily activities. *Journal of Speech, Language, and Hearing Research, 44*(3), 511–524. https://doi.org/10.1044/1092–4388(2001/040)

Magee, M., Lewis, C., Noffs, G., Reece, H., Chan, J. C. S., Zaga, C. J., . . . Vogel, A. P. (2020). Effects of face masks on acoustic analysis and speech perception: Implications for peri–pandemic protocols. *The Journal of the Acoustical Society of America, 148*(6), 3562–3568. https://doi.org/10.1121/10.0002873

Maryn, Y., & Zarowski, A. J. (2015). Calibration of clinical audio recording and analysis aystems for aound intensity measurement. *American Journal of Speech–Language Pathology, 24*(4), 608–618. https://doi.org/10.1044/2015_AJSLP–14–0082

Myers, B., Hary, E., Ellerston, J., & Barkmeier-Kraemer, J. (2022). Telepractice considerations for evaluation and treatment of voice disorders: Tailoring to specific populations. *American Journal of Speech–Language Pathology,* 1–11. ePub ahead of issue. *https://doi.org/10.1044/2021_AJSLP–21–00206*

Patel, R. (2002). Prosodic control in severe dysarthria: Preserved ability to mark the question-statement contrast. *Journal of Speech, Language, and Hearing Research, 45*(5), 858–870. https://doi.org/10.1044/1092–4388(2002/069)

Patel, R. (2011). Assessment of prosody. In A. Lowit & R. D. Kent (Eds.), *Assessment of motor speech disorders* (pp. 75–96). Plural Publishing.

Patel, R., Awan, S., Barkmeier-Kraemer, J., Courey, M., Deliyski, D., Eadie, T., . . . Hillman, R. (2018). Recommended protocols for instrumental assessment of voice: American speech-language-hearing association expert panel to develop a protocol for instrumental assessment of vocal function. *American Journal of Speech-Language Pathology 27*(3), 887–905. https://doi.org/10.1044/2018_AJSLP–17–0009

Patel, R., & Campellone, P. (2009). Acoustic and perceptual cues to contrastive stress in dysarthria. *Journal of Speech, Language, and Hearing Research, 52*(1), 206–222. https://doi.org/10.1044/1092–4388(2008/07–0078)

Paul, D. R., Frattali, C. M., Holland, A. L., Thompson, C. K., Caperton, C. J., & Slater, S. C. (2004). *American Speech–Language–Hearing Association Quality of Communication Life Scale (AHSA QCL): Manual.* American Speech-Language-Hearing Association.

Robertson, S. J., & Thomson, F. (1987). *Working with dysarthric clients: A practical guide to therapy for dysarthria.* Communication Skill Builders.

Rosen, C. A., Lee, A. S., Osborne, J., Zullo, T., & Murry, T. (2004). Development and validation of the Voice Handicap Index–10. *The Laryngoscope, 114*(9), 1549–1556. https://doi.org/10.1097/00005537–200409000–00009

Sapienza, C., & Hoffman, B. (2022). *Voice disorders* (4th ed.). Plural Publishing.

Schneider, S. L., Habich, L., Weston, Z. M., & Rosen, C. A. (2021). Observations and considerations for implementing remote acoustic voice recording and analysis in clinical practice. *Journal of Voice* [Advance online publication]. https://doi.org/10.1016/j.jvoice.2021.06.011

Snyder, C., Jensen., R., Segal, J., & Wu., A. (2013). Patient–reported outcomes (PROs): Putting the patient perspective in patient–centered outcomes research. *Medical Care, 51*(8), S73–S79. http://www.doi.org/10.1097/MLR.0b013e31829b1d84

Stemple, J. C., Roy, N., & Klaben, B. K. (2014). *Clinical voice pathology: Theory and management* (5th ed.). Plural Publishing.

Strand, E. A., Duffy, J. R., Clark, H. M., & Josephs, K. (2014). The apraxia of speech rating scale: A tool for diagnosis and description of apraxia of speech. *Journal of Communication Disorders, 51*, 43–50. https://doi.org/10.1016/j.jcomdis.2014.06.008

Švec, J. G., & Granqvist, S. (2018). Tutorial and guidelines on measurement of sound pressure level in voice and speech. *Journal of Speech, Language, and Hearing Research 61*(3), 441–461. https://doi.org/10.1044/2017_JSLHR–S–17–0095

Swigert, N. B. (2010). *The source for dysarthria* (2nd ed.). Pro–Ed.

Vos, T. G., Dillon, M. T., Buss, E., Rooth, M. A., Bucker, A. L., Dillon, S., . . . Dedmon, M. M. 2021), Influence of protective face coverings on the speech recognition of cochlear implant patients. *The Laryngoscope, 131*, E2038–E2043. https://doi.org/10.1002/lary.29447

Walshe, M., Peach, R. K., & Miller, N. (2009). Dysarthria Impact Profile: Development of a scale to measure psychosocial effects. *International Journal of Language & Communication Disorders, 44*(5), 693–715. https://doi.org/10.1080/13682820802317536

World Health Organization. (2001). *International classification of functioning, disability, and health.* https://www.who.int/standards/classifications/international–classification–of–functioning–disability–and–health

Yorkston, K., & Baylor, C. (2019). Patient–reported outcomes measures: An introduction for clinicians. *Perspectives of the ASHA Special Interest Groups, 4*(1), 8–15. https://doi.org/10.1044/2018_PERS–ST–2018–0001

Zraick, R. I., Risner, B. Y., Smith–Olinde, L., Gregg, B. A., Johnson, F. L., & McWeeny, E. K. (2007). Patient versus partner perception of voice handicap. *Journal of Voice, 21*(4) 485–494. https://doi.org/10.1016/j.jvoice.2006.06.006

APPENDIX 3–1

Communicative Effectiveness Survey-Revised (CESR)

Name: _____ Date: _____

Responder (please circle):   **Self**   **Communication Partner**

Instructions: Self: For each statement below, please circle the number that reflects how effectively you communicate in each situation (1=not at all effective to 4=very effective).
Communication Partner: For each statement below, please circle the number that reflects how effectively your communication partner communicates in each situation (1=not at all effective to 4=very effective).

		1	2	3	4
1.	Communicating your wants and needs to a family member at home.	1	2	3	4
2.	Having a conversation with family members or friends at home.	1	2	3	4
3.	Having a conversation with a familiar person over the telephone.	1	2	3	4
4.	Having a conversation outdoors in a quiet environment (for example a café).	1	2	3	4
5.	Having a conversation with a health care provider.	1	2	3	4
6.	Talking in person to service people (for example, a bank teller or a waiter).	1	2	3	4
7.	Exchanging greetings with someone.	1	2	3	4
8.	Having a long conversation with another couple at home.	1	2	3	4
9.	Speaking when you are excited about or interested in the topic.	1	2	3	4
10.	Calling for help to someone in another part of the house or outside.	1	2	3	4
11.	Having a conversation with a young child.	1	2	3	4

		1	2	3	4
12.	Talking over the phone to service people (for example, plumber, phone company).	1	2	3	4
13.	Having a conversation while riding as a passenger in a car.	1	2	3	4
14.	Participating in conversations with a small group of people (for example, several couples over dinner).	1	2	3	4
15.	Engaging in small talk with someone you've just met.	1	2	3	4
16.	Communicating your wants and needs to a family member away from home.	1	2	3	4
17.	Speaking when you are angry.	1	2	3	4
18.	Entering into an ongoing conversation.	1	2	3	4
19.	Communicating with someone who is in the next room.	1	2	3	4
20.	Talking in person with someone who has an unfamiliar accent.	1	2	3	4
21.	Having a conversation when it's hard for you to hear.	1	2	3	4
22.	Having a conversation with someone who is hard of hearing.	1	2	3	4
23.	Speaking when you are emotionally upset.	1	2	3	4
24.	Having a conversation indoors in a noisy environment (for example, a social gathering).	1	2	3	4
25.	Talking over the telephone with someone who has an unfamiliar accent.	1	2	3	4
26.	Having a conversation when you are tired or fatigued.	1	2	3	4
27.	Having a conversation outdoors in a noisy environment (for example, a football game or big social gathering).	1	2	3	4
	TOTAL RAW SCORE: Transfer to the CESR Score Conversion Chart (see next page)				

© **Neila J. Donovan, PhD, CCC-SLP COMMUNICATIVE EFFECTIVE-NESS SURVEY REVISED (CESR)**
Louisiana State University Department of Communication Sciences and Disorders ndonovan@lsu.edu

LSU	COMMUNICATIVE EFFECTIVENESS SURVEY-Revised© (CESR)RAW SCORE TO 0-100 INTERVAL SCORE	

NAME: _____

DATE:_____   **Total Raw Score =**_____   **Scale Score =** _____

Directions:
1. Enter Name.
2. Enter Date.
3. Enter Total Raw Score from Response Form in the appropriate space.
4. Locate Total Raw Score on Table below in the left-most column.
5. Move one column to the right to find the Scale Score. Enter Scale Score in the space provided.

TOTAL RAW SCORE	SCALE SCORE	S.E.	TOTAL RAW SCORE	SCALE SCORE	S.E.	TOTAL RAW SCORE	SCALE SCORE	S.E.
29	0	12.7	56	40	2.05	82	56	2.2
30	9	7.1	57	41	2.04	83	57	2.2
31	14	5.1	58	41	2.03	84	57	2.2
32	17	4.3	59	42	2.02	85	58	2.2
33	19	3.8	60	43	2.02	86	59	2.3
34	21	3.5	61	43	2.01	87	60	2.3
35	23	3.2	62	44	2.01	88	60	2.3
36	24	3.0	63	44	2.01	89	61	2.4
37	25	2.9	64	45	2.01	90	62	2.4
38	27	2.8	65	46	2.01	91	63	2.5
39	28	2.7	66	46	2.01	92	64	2.5
40	29	2.6	67	47	2.01	93	65	2.6
41	30	2.5	68	47	2.01	94	66	2.6
42	30	2.4	69	48	2.02	95	67	2.7
43	31	2.4	70	48	2.02	96	68	2.8
44	32	2.3	71	49	2.03	97	69	2.9
45	33	2.3	72	50	2.03	98	70	3.0
46	34	2.3	73	50	2.04	99	72	3.1
47	34	2.2	74	51	2.05	100	73	3.3
48	35	2.2	75	52	2.06	101	75	3.5
49	36	2.2	76	52	2.07	102	77	3.8
50	36	2.2	77	53	2.08	103	79	4.1
51	37	2.1	78	53	2.1	104	82	4.6
52	38	2.1	79	54	2.11	105	85	5.5
53	38	2.1	80	55	2.13	106	91	7.3
54	39	2.1	81	55	2.14	107	100	12.8
55	40	2.1						

Reproduced with permission from Neila J. Donovan.

APPENDIX 3–2

The Communicative Participation Item Bank—General Short Form

Instructions:

The following questions describe a variety of situations in which you might need to speak to others. For each question, please mark how much your condition interferes with your participation in that situation. By "condition" we mean ALL issues that may affect how you communicate in these situations including speech conditions, any other health conditions, or features of the environment. If your speech varies, think about an AVERAGE day for your speech – not your best or your worst days.

	Not at all (3)	A little (2)	Quite a bit (1)	Very much (0)
1. Does your condition interfere with... **...talking with people you know?**	O	O	O	O
2. Does your condition interfere with... **...communicating when you need to say something quickly?**	O	O	O	O
3. Does your condition interfere with... **...talking with people you do NOT know?**	O	O	O	O

	Not at all (3)	A little (2)	Quite a bit (1)	Very much (0)
4. Does your condition interfere with... **...communicating when you are out in your community (e.g. errands; appointments)?**	○	○	○	○
5. Does your condition interfere with... **...asking questions in a conversation?**	○	○	○	○
6. Does your condition interfere with... **...communicating in a small group of people?**	○	○	○	○
7. Does your condition interfere with... **...having a long conversation with someone you know about a book, movie, show or sports event?**	○	○	○	○
8. Does your condition interfere with... **... giving someone DETAILED information?**	○	○	○	○

	Not at all (3)	A little (2)	Quite a bit (1)	Very much (0)
9. Does your condition interfere with... **...getting your turn in a fast-moving conversation?**	○	○	○	○
10. Does your condition interfere with... **...trying to persuade a friend or family member to see a different point of view?**	○	○	○	○

SCORING GUIDE FOR THE CPIB GENERAL SHORT FORM

To score the short form, add the scores for the ten items to obtain a summary score (Not at all = 3; A little = 2; Quite a bit = 1; Very much = 0). The summary score will range from 0 – 30. High scores are more favorable, meaning that high scores indicate less interference in participation. Using the table below, the summary scores can be converted to IRT theta values (logit scale). On the logit scale, scores generally range from -3.0 to +3.0 with 0 logits representing the mean for the calibration sample. Again, high scores are preferable. The table also includes a conversion to standard T scores (mean = 50; standard deviation = 10). **VERY IMPORTANT: This score translation table is ONLY valid for the 10 item short form presented in this manuscript.** Remember that in IRT, the person score is based on the parameters of the individual items and on how the person answers the items. This scoring table has been generated using the item parameters for the ten items in this short form, and these parameters would differ for different items. A new score translation table must be created for any other combination of items.

CPIB 10-Item General Short Form Scoring Table						
Summary	Theta	T score		Summary	Theta	T score
0	−2.58	24.20		16	-0.22	47.80
1	−2.18	28.20		17	-0.10	49.00
2	−1.94	30.60		18	0.03	50.30
3	−1.76	32.40		19	0.15	51.50
4	−1.60	34.00		20	0.27	52.70
5	−1.46	35.40		21	0.40	54.00
6	−1.34	36.60		22	0.53	55.30
7	−1.22	37.80		23	0.65	56.50
8	−1.10	39.00		24	0.78	57.80
9	−0.99	40.10		25	0.92	59.20
10	−0.89	41.10		26	1.06	60.60
11	−0.78	42.20		27	1.22	62.20
12	−0.67	43.30		28	1.42	64.20
13	−0.56	44.40		29	1.67	66.70
14	−0.45	45.50		30	2.10	71.00
15	−0.33	46.70				

Baylor, C., Yorkston, K., Eadie, T., Kim, J., Chung, H., & Amtmann, D. (2013). The Communicative Participation Item Bank (CPIB): Item bank calibration and development of a disorder-generic short form. *Journal of Speech Language and Hearing Research, 56*, 1190–1208.

Website for downloading this short form or administering the CPIB via computerized adaptive testing:
http://depts.washington.edu/cpib
(*Note:* This website does not store any PHI. It actually does not store any data so write down your scores.)

Contact: Carolyn Baylor at cbaylor@uw.edu

CHAPTER 4

Factors Related to Meaningful Assessment of Intelligibility

Key Points:

- Many SLPs believe intelligibility measures are important but they reported limited access to and use of formal measures.

- Factors related to the speaker, such as severity, rate, fatigue, and motivation level can influence measures of intelligibility.

- The type of message the client speaks can impact an intelligibility score if the message is predictable or familiar to the listener.

- If the listener receives auditory and visual information as opposed to only auditory, intelligibility scores can be affected. Care should be taken to understand whether the visual information helps listeners understand the message or not.

- Factors related to listeners, including experience with the speech disorder, familiarity with the speaker or message, and age can impact intelligibility measures.

- To obtain comparable pre- and post-treatment measures, SLPs should keep factors related to the speaker, message, listener, and communication environment consistent across intelligibility assessments.

This chapter focuses on examination of challenges related to activities and participation, focusing specifically on measurement of a speaker's intelligibility. Consideration of the ICF (World Health Organization, 2001) model areas of activity and participation limitations allows us to include the functional aspects that may keep our clients from feeling like successful communicators. When we examine successful communication, we want to be sure we are including both communicators and the environment. Years of research have taught us that factors related to the speaker, the listener and how the message is sent can influence intelligibility measures. Schiavetti (1992) points out that if you want to measure intelligibility in a disordered speaker, you will want to control or keep constant the influences of the listener and the "transmission" system, such as signal-to-noise ratio. Research in our field has taught us about how factors related to the speaker and the message can affect intelligibility measures. If we know what these are, we can attempt to keep them constant to allow for some level of comparison between measures. If you want to compare baseline measures with those following a period of treatment, you want to be sure you are comparing consistent measures. Selection of the message used in intelligibility assessment can also influence assessment and suggestions will be described in this chapter, related to research findings.

CLINICIAN'S USE AND PERCEPTIONS
OF INTELLIGIBILITY MEASURES

Most textbooks and resources about dysarthria stress that reduced intelligibility is a key functional limitation in clients with dysarthria and an important clinical target (Duffy, 2019; Lowit & Kent, 2011; Swigert, 2010). A survey of SLPs who work with patients with dysarthria found that 93% of those surveyed felt intelligibility was an important measure in their assessment and management (Miller et al., 2011). Many SLPs working with clients with dysarthria do not use standardized procedures to assess intelligibility (Collis & Bloch, 2012; Gurevich & Scamihorn, 2017; King et al., 2012; Miller et al., 2011). Reasons for not using formal assessments included limitations on time, funding, and available resources. SLPs also mentioned they were not satisfied with standardized assessments or did not have knowledge of them. Limited time or knowledge about using intelligibility measures can lead to even more ineffective use of clinicians' resources. Using assessment to clearly identify the issues contributing to a client's reduced intelligibility can lead to selection of proper targets for therapy and the ability to compare measures over time to document progress. Gurevich and Scamihorn (2017) noted a trend that even SLPs who reported having access to standardized assessment protocols preferred using informal methods. In fact, many SLPs reported they find oral mechanism exams, diadochokinetic measures, and cranial nerve exams to be simple, effective, and useful ways to measure intelligibility (Gurevich & Scamihorn, 2017; Miller et al., 2011). These three examples do not provide a measure of speech, let alone intelligibility. Measures such as oral mechanism exams, diadochokinetic measures, and cranial nerve exams give information related to movements and sensation of the oral structures. These measures do not provide information related to intelligibility because we do not learn anything about how a listener handles the auditory information. The studies mentioned here concluded that responses reflected potential needs for new assessment procedures, as well as further training and education for SLPs. This chapter provides findings from studies on intelligibility that can help guide your functional assessment of your client's activity limitations and participation restrictions.

INTELLIGIBILITY ASSESSMENT

A holistic approach that looks at the whole person is the best way for an SLP to learn as much as possible about a client's communicative effectiveness. Researchers often refer to the "top down" perspective, which here means we are considering all aspects of how the client communicates in a real-life environment. This approach allows us to avoid a "bottom up" perspective which involves measuring all of the small details that contribute to the client's communication.

Using a holistic approach will include gathering information about interactions with different communicative partners and communication environments. It can take a great deal of time to gather information to have a holistic view of a client. An initial measure of intelligibility will provide a starting point for qualifying a client for services, a baseline measure of the severity of impairment, and a direction for the management chosen (Gurevich & Scamihorn, 2017). If the goal is to help listeners understand the speaker, then a measure of intelligibility is critical. There are many factors related to how you measure your client's intelligibility that will affect the outcome. Using what we've learned from research studies can help us gain useful information about our client's intelligibility. Stating that a client is "80% intelligible" provides very little detail as to what message they sent, who the listener was, and what the communication environment was. For this reason, Hustad and Weismer (2007) suggest that when we make that type of statement, we consider that the measure applies only to the speaker with a particular listener, in a specific environment, using a particular message that they refer to as a " . . . snapshot of speech adequacy at a moment in time on a particular set of stimuli with a particular set of listeners" (p. 266). We can categorize intelligibility measures as objective or subjective, depending on the tasks used (Yorkston & Beukelman, 1978), and knowing each type of measure involved will help you decide which is best for your client.

Subjective Intelligibility Measurement Tasks

When we use subjective measures, we ask listeners to assign a number or percentage that equates to their perception of a speaker's intelligibility. We can use these ratings with different speaker messages, including samples taken from conversational speech, sentences that are read, or responses to questions. Schiavetti (1992) describes the use of equal-appearing interval (EAI) scales, which is one type of subjective measure. When using EAI scales, listeners are asked to choose a number that best characterizes the speech sample when given a linear interval scale with a range (e.g., 1 to 5). Descriptor words can identify the points on the far ends of the scale (i.e., 1 = totally unintelligible; 5 = totally intelligible). Another strategy for subjective intelligibility measurement is use of a percentage estimate. Listeners hear a speech sample and then estimate the percentage of words they understood on a scale ranging from 0 to 100 (Schiavetti, 1992; Yorkston & Beukelman, 1978).

There are pros and cons to using these scaling procedures for subjective measurement of intelligibility (Metz et al., 1980). The scales could be developed and used easily and inexpensively, as there is no test or equipment required. A primary concern is that there is subjectivity in the actual scaling where one person may scale differently than another. Miller (2013) described how listeners have their own individual "internal yardstick" to measure, which results in a lack of agreement during ratings. These types of measures may tell you that your client's intelligibility is reduced but don't provide any detail about what to target in treatment.

Objective Intelligibility Measurement Tasks

We usually complete objective intelligibility measures by having listeners transcribe words or sentences. This may take place online, at the time of the evaluation, with the SLP serving as the transcriber as specified in directions of the Frenchay Dysarthria Test—Second Edition (Enderby & Palmer, 2008). But, in most cases, the transcriber or listener will not be the clinician and the speaker will be audio recorded so the sample can be played at a later time. Refer to the information in Chapter 3 on factors that affect our recording of speech samples. The listener should not know what the speech stimuli or message is. We can count the number of words that are correctly transcribed to obtain an intelligibility score. Some researchers who study the measurement of intelligibility have adapted rules for acceptable responses to include minor morphological errors, including tense difference, spelling errors, and homophones, as long as the syllable structure is intact (Fontan et al., 2015; Hustad & Cahill, 2003; Liss et al., 2000; Borrie et al., 2019). You can obtain an intelligibility percentage score by dividing the number of words correctly transcribed by the total number of words possible and then multiplying by 100 (Tikofsky & Tikofsky, 1964; Yorkston & Beukelman, 1978). Most formal intelligibility measures use this method, including the Assessment of the Intelligibility of Dysarthric Speech (AIDS; Yorkston & Beukelman, 1984), and the Sentence Intelligibility Test (SIT; Yorkston et al., 2007). Transcription is considered the clinical gold standard because it allows us to take a quantitative measure of what listeners perceive (Hustad & Weismer, 2007). Table 4–1 contains descriptions and information on how to obtain tools for evaluation of intelligibility. When selecting a method to measure intelligibility, it is helpful to consider what you want to learn in your assessment. If you want to quantify or have a percentage to describe a client's intelligibility, the AIDS and SIT will provide you with that information using a standardized format. If you want to know specific articulatory targets for management, the Multi-Word Intelligibility Test (MWIT; Kent et al., 1989) can help you determine which errors are contributing to the client's reduced intelligibility.

Rather than purchasing a formal intelligibility test, SLPs can use word or sentence lists created to measure intelligibility in different populations. Table 4–1 contains several examples of word or sentence lists and information on accessing those lists. Use the information provided in this table to help you decide for each client which formal tool or list of sentences might be most useful. For example, if you would like to measure intelligibility and speech rate, the AIDS or SIT might be useful tools to consider. You may work with a client whose facial movements may be noticeable or distracting. In this case, to determine a functional, real-world measure that captures the impact of the visual information, you may select the Medical Research Council (MRC) Institute of Hearing Research (MacLeod & Summerfield, 1990) audiovisual sentence lists that were created to control for impact of visual information. These lists are provided for your use in Appendix 4–1. If you wanted to evaluate how listeners' perception is affected by this type of client, you can show the listeners videos, rather than just using audio recordings. You can see that there are a lot of choices, so be aware that using a measure at baseline and a different measure after treatment won't allow you to compare scores. This will vary between different measures and can be influenced by different severities of impairment. Hustad (2006) found that transcription scores were higher than percentage estimate, but the amount of difference varied between the speakers.

Table 4–1. Instruments and Materials for Assessment of Intelligibility in Adults

Instrument, Authors, Year Published, How to Access	Stimuli or Message	Listener, Task, and Mode of Presentation
Word Intelligibility Lists Tikofsky & Tikofsky (1964) https://doi.org/10.1044/jshr.0704.325	■ 50 CVC words ■ 50 randomly selected spondee words (words with 2 equally stressed syllables, e.g., "Wildcat") ■ 60 monosyllabic words with initial and final clusters	■ Audio recording ■ Measured by listener transcription ■ Score is obtained by the number of words correctly identified.
Single Word Intelligibility Test Tikofsky (1970) https://doi.org/10.1044/jshr.1301.59	■ 50 monosyllabic or bisyllabic words	■ Audio recording ■ Measured by listener transcription ■ Score is obtained by the number of words correctly identified.
Phonetically Balanced Single-Word Test Platt, Andrews, Young, & Quinn (1980) https://doi.org/10.1044/jshr.2301.28	■ 50 phonetically balanced words ■ Grandfather passage reading	■ Audio Recording ■ Words measured by listener transcription ■ Reading passage rated with 7-point scale ("not understandable to understandable")

Test		

Assessment of Intelligibility of Dysarthric Speech (AIDS)
 	
Yorkston & Beukelman (1984)
 	
https://www.proedaust.com.au/assessment-of-intelligibility-of-dysarthric-speech-aids
	■ 50 randomly selected words (from large pool of phonetically similar words)
	
	■ select 2 at each sentence length (from 5 to 15 words) from more than 1000 sentences
		■ Audio Recording
		■ Multiple choice word test with target words and three foils
		OR
		■ Listener transcription of words or sentences
		■ Score is percentage of words correctly identified
		■ Provides related measures
		  □ Speaking rate
		  □ Rate of intelligible speech
		  □ Rate of unintelligible speech
		■ Communication efficiency ratio

Multi-Word Intelligibility Test (MWIT) Kent, Weismer, Kent, & Rosenbek (1989) https://doi.org/10.1044/jshd.5404.482	■ 70 words with 19 minimal phonetic contrasts sets of words (sip, ship, tip, zip) ■ 48 words of CV or VC syllables for more severe clients ■ There are 3 words pairs for each of 16 phonetic contrasts (shoe, chew)	■ Audio Recording ■ Multiple choice word test with target word and three foils ■ Paired words test – listener selects one ■ Both versions allow the clinician to determine which phonemes may have the most impact on intelligibility

continues

Table 4–1. *continued*

Instrument, Authors, Year Published, How to Access	Stimuli or Message	Listener, Task, and Mode of Presentation
Medical Research Council (MRC) Institute of Hearing Research Audio-Visual Sentence Lists MacLeod & Summerfield (1990) See Appendix 4–1	■ 10 sets of 15 sentences equalized for lipreading and presence of visibly distinct consonants containing equal number of sentences with the same syntactic structure (e.g., subject-verb-object). ■ MRC lists 2 to 8 and 10 were found to have low predictability (between 19% to 28%) Keintz, Bunton & Hoit (2007)	■ Developed for speech in noise tests Bench et al. (1979)
Hearing in Noise Test Nilsson, Soli, & Sullivan (1994) See Appendix 4–2	■ Set of 25 lists of 10 phonemically balanced sentences each	■ Developed to test speech reception threshold in quiet and in noise
Unpredictable Sentences for Intelligibility Testing McHenry & Parle (2006) https://www.researchgate.net /publication/328570024 _Construction_of_a_set_of _unpredictable_sentences_for _intelligibility_testing	■ Set of 50, 7-word sentences designed so that words are relatively unpredictable	■ Directions for use are not stated but the list was developed for us by clinicians. ■ Lack of predictability is suggested to ensure evaluation of intelligibility rather than comprehensibility.

Sentence Intelligibility Test for Windows (SIT) Yorkston, Beukelman, Hakel, & Dorsey (2007) https://www.madonna.org/institute/software	■ Computerized test through Windows ■ Words ■ Sentences—program selects 11 (short version) or 22 sentences from a pool of 1100 that range from 5 to 15 words	■ Audio Recording ■ Hard copy or computerized versions available ■ Words—listener selects from 6 choices to identify ■ Listener transcription of sentences ■ Score is percentage of words correctly identified ■ Provides related measures 　□ Speaking rate 　□ Rate of intelligible speech 　□ Rate of unintelligible speech ■ Communication efficiency ratio
Frenchay Dysarthria Assessment (Second edition) FDA-2 Enderby & Palmer (2008) Available for purchase from: (1) Pro-Ed. https://www.proedinc.com/Products/12685/fda2-frenchay-dysarthria-assessmentsecond-edition.aspx (2) Pearson https://www.pearsonclinical.com.au/products/view/485	■ SLP selects10 words from a pool of 116 words ■ SLP selects 10 short sentences from a pool of 50 sentences ranging from 2 to 6 words ■ 5-minute conversational sample	■ Online/live clinician transcription OR ■ Audio record clinician transcription ■ Words & sentences rated on a 5-point scale to reflect difference in number of words correctly recognized or ease of word recognition. ■ Conversational sample rated on a 5-point severity scale ranging from "no abnormality" to "totally unintelligible"

continues

Table 4–1. *continued*

Instrument, Authors, Year Published, How to Access	Stimuli or Message	Listener, Task, and Mode of Presentation
Chapel Hill Multilingual Intelligibility Test	■ Designed to use with computer software for PC and Mac	■ Audio Recording
https://www.med.unc.edu/ahs /sphs/card/resources/chapel-hill -multilingual-intelligibility-test-chmit/	■ Software available free of cost— for permission, email card@med. unc.edu.	■ Measured by listener transcription
Languages Available:	■ 50 sets of 12 monosyllabic words	■ One word from each set is randomly selected by the software
English Haley (2011)		■ Speakers hears a model and repeats (no reading).
Swedish Gery & Haley (2011)		■ Test administrator does not need to know the language tested.
Russian Dolgova & Haley (2011)		■ Listener must be fluent in tested language
Hindi Salaria & Haley (2011)		
German Thiessen & Haley (2011)		
French Jozefowicz & Haley (2011)		
Finnish Morris & Haley (2011)		
Spanish Fischer & Haley (2014)		
Greek Pravasilis & Haley (2014)		
Danish Gammelgaard & Haley (2016)		

INFLUENCES ON INTELLIGIBILITY MEASURES

Years of research have demonstrated that there are many factors that can influence the results of intelligibility measures. Knowing about these factors and controlling for them when possible will help ensure the accuracy of your intelligibility measures. This chapter introduces factors that can influence intelligibility measures related to the speaker and the message. Factors related to the listener and communication environment should also be considered and are covered in later chapters.

Factors Related to the Speaker

Among adults who have reduced intelligibility, there will be various etiologies and severities that will cause them to look and sound different from each other. The focus of this book is individuals with dysarthria, apraxia of speech, and voice disorders, including alaryngeal speech. Disorder type, in itself, could be a factor. First, even within one disorder, such as dysarthria, there are seven dysarthria types, all with different perceptual characteristics (Duffy, 2019). There are even more types of voice disorders, so it is safe to say that among the adults with reduced intelligibility in a clinician's caseload, there will be a very heterogeneous group. Many studies have revealed differences in intelligibility between speakers with different etiologies or dysarthria types (Klasner & Yorkston, 2005; Liss et al., 2000; Stipancic et al., 2016). Second, the etiology can vary in this population and change the course of progression. Hustad and Weismer (2007) discuss etiologies that are improving, degenerating, and chronic or stable. When determining how best to measure intelligibility, etiology progression may be an important consideration. For example, in measuring intelligibility in an individual with a degenerating disease process like ALS, when you move from a baseline measure to a post-treatment measure, you are likely assessing the impact of treatment along with the progression of this disease. In some cases, following a stroke, you might see improvement related to spontaneous recovery, alongside gains made in treatment. It's important to consider all likely factors related to your client's abilities when comparing pre/post treatment measures. If you are completing a baseline assessment, you may want to simply determine the client's natural state. Clients may have learned strategies either in previous therapy or on their own that enhance their intelligibility. Figure 1–1 in Chapter 1 reminds us that the compensations by speakers related to rate, effort, and phrasing contribute to the acoustic signal or what speakers hear. If you want to learn if a client's intelligibility has changed after treatment or during disease progression, you may want to consider taking a measure while asking the client to utilize strategies they have learned. As you can see, considering all of these choices will lead to a client-specific assessment plan. Factors related specifically to the speaker will be discussed here so you can use what we've learned from research to drive your decision-making.

Severity

Many studies of intelligibility examine different severity levels when they compare speaker performances. Research has shown that intelligibility scores vary based on severity; severity also interacts with other study variables in most cases (Yorkston & Beukelman, 1978; Hustad & Cahill, 2003; Keintz et al., 2007). When reading research, it is helpful to understand how investigators are defining "severity." Researchers may use an overall severity of the dysarthria, or severity may be related to the intelligibility itself. If we use terms like "mild," "moderate," and "severe," there is no standard directive in the field as to what intelligibility level falls into each of these categories. Because severity is analyzed in such a large number of intelligibility studies, it is a good idea to be sure you consider the severity level of your clients when determining evaluation and management that is most appropriate for their needs and abilities.

Speech Rate

Quite a few studies have examined the impact of different techniques to slow the rate of speech on intelligibility. There have been inconsistent findings, but it is important to note that changing rate of speech can affect intelligibility measures. Some studies have found that slowing rate improves intelligibility (Hammen et al., 1994; Turner et al., 1995; Yorkston et al., 1990). Other studies have not found consistently that slowing rate improves intelligibility (McAuliffe et al., 2014; Tjaden & Wilding, 2004). Many of the differences related to rate reduction in these and other studies are likely due to different dysarthria types of these individuals. The studies mentioned previously had several etiologies in the study population, including cerebral palsy, Parkinson's disease, and multiple sclerosis. Another factor is that studies often use different strategies to reduce rate. The important point to remember on this topic when completing an intelligibility assessment is that rate can influence your measure. Some clients may have learned rate reduction strategies on their own or through previous therapy, so you won't be able to control for rate in all instances. When taking a baseline measure of intelligibility, the optimal way to address this is to ask the client to use normal, everyday speech. You may want to take post-treatment measures that examine the rate, so that in those instances, you can direct the client to use strategies you've instructed them to use. Remember, their performance may be influenced by what you ask them to do, so think about the instructions you give clients when asking them to read or speak the messages you will use to measure intelligibility. Using consistent instructions will allow you to have a similar protocol between clients or between measures of the same client, which will increase the reliability of your measures.

Personal Speaker Factors

If you are measuring a baseline or taking a follow-up measure after treatment, there are other factors to consider. The main consideration is to be as consistent as possible with these issues, which may not be in your control or even the client's. If you are working with a client who experiences fatigue, aim to record the speaker when they are at their best. Keep in mind though, that they have reduced intelligibility when they feel fatigued. Ideally, we would record the client when they are feeling motivated to take part. Some clients will take medications that may have peaks in their cycles. A client who is taking medication for Parkinson's disease is a good example, as those medications tend to have on/off effects. A medication cycle for this patient may include time when the medication causes too much movement or too little movement, which could influence intelligibility measures. Consider whether it is useful for you to know how the client sounds when medication is most effective versus when it is not. At the very least, you should gather information on when they last took their medication, so you can consider this when you interpret the results of assessment. If you keep the medication timing the same on pre-treatment versus post-treatment data, you will reduce the effect of medication on your results. Some of these clients will have co-occurring disturbances in sensation, cognition, language, hearing, or other areas. Plan your tasks for the speaker accordingly. It is important to give thought to the speaker factors that can influence intelligibility scores, so if you are measuring to baseline or examine for change over time, that you are truly getting a comparable measure that is not influenced by other factors.

Factors Related to the Message

Measuring intelligibility of our clients in their most everyday, natural circumstances might feel like the most functional way to do this. The type of message that we ask our speakers to produce can have an influence on the intelligibility measurement, so it's a good idea to know what these factors are and how we can work around them.

Type of Message

Consider what you want to learn about your client's intelligibility when you select the stimulus or message. This is a complex issue because speaker factors, such as severity, will play a role. Speakers with more mild levels of dysarthria had higher intelligibility scores on sentences compared to words (Hustad, 2007; Yorkston & Beukelman, 1978, 1981). When this happens, listeners are probably taking advantage of the context of the other words in the sentence, which they may understand in a speaker whose intelligibility is not severely reduced. However, for speakers in the moderate-to-severe levels of dysarthria, no differences were found between word and sentence intelligibility (Hustad, 2007). In contrast to those studies, a recent study showed lower intelligibility scores from words in sentences than in isolated words with no pattern related to speaker severity (Barreto & Ortiz, 2020). Patel and colleagues (2014) found that in speakers with various dysarthria types and severities resulted in similar intelligibility scores between words and sentences. But, when these researchers pulled out words that were produced in sentences and presented them in isolation, there was a decrease in intelligibility levels of those words. This might mean that speaking at sentence level may result in using less articulation clarity. That makes sense if we consider that fatigue is an issue with many of our clients with reduced intelligibility. Longer sentences may be harder to produce and therefore less intelligible but, in some cases, listeners are gaining information from context. There are many issues to consider and each client's situation, even with various listeners may call for a different plan to maximize intelligibility. Appendix 4–2 contains sentences from the Hearing in Noise Test (Nilsson et al., 1994), which was developed to be equalized in length, difficulty, and phonemic distribution. As there are 25 lists containing ten sentences each, SLPs could use different lists for pre and posttreatment intelligibility assessment.

Although research results are not totally consistent regarding words/sentences, your choice of stimuli may be determined by how severely your client's intelligibility is reduced. More severe speakers may not have high intelligibility at sentence levels and not show differences between very low scores if you are comparing pre/posttreatment measures. For less severe clients, intelligibility may be very high and again not show differences at the single word level. Using single words will not show you about the client's prosody or longer speech sequences, which can be reasons for reduced intelligibility that you may miss. If possible, it would be helpful to assess using both single words and sentences to give you the broadest picture of your client's communication skills. If you find your client is more intelligible with single words than multiword utterances, this helps you know that when you teach your client how to handle communication breakdowns, single-word utterances will be useful. Or, if intelligibility is higher at sentence level, you know listeners are probably using contextual information and that might be the most effective way for the client to communicate.

Beyond word and sentence levels, you could consider using a paragraph reading, which allows for some control over what is read but isn't truly conversational. This might allow you to have a longer representation of the client's connected speech but still know what words they are reading. Two reading passages are commonly used in speech assessments, Grandfather Passage (Van Riper, 1963) and the Rainbow Passage (Fairbanks, 1960).

Both are easily accessible by doing an Internet search. Using a conversational sample may seem like the most natural and functional choice. However, if you do not have a reliable key to what the client said, your ability to score words as correct or not will not be accurate. In conversation, you are not able to control for syntax, semantics, and the phonemes that are produced. When you plan how to measure intelligibility, you can use your best judgment given your client's needs and abilities. If you plan to compare scores directly, you will want to use consistent types of messages. But using the same sentences with the same listener may lead to them remembering the sentences. Word and sentence lists, like those lists in Table 4–1, are useful because they represent similar but not identical messages.

Predictability of Message

You might not have thought about the predictability of sentences before, but you should consider this when you select sentences for intelligibility measures. Studies of intelligibility have examined the impact of syntactic and semantic predictability. Syntactic predictability occurs when sentences contain a high level of grammatical predictiveness. In English, this could be as structured as subject, verb, object (e.g., He reads a book). Sentences that have highly predictable syntax resulted in higher intelligibility compared to those with low predictable syntax in speakers with dysarthria (Carter et al., 1996). Semantic predictability refers to the fact that you may miss a word in a particular sentence, but you can "guess" the word or fill in the blank because the rest of the sentence provides contextual cues. If we use the example sentence suggested earlier to be syntactically predictable, "He reads a book," we could alter it to be less predictable by substituting the verb "owns" instead of "reads." It still makes sense semantically to say, "He owns a book," but it is less predictable. If a listener is writing what they hear, but they do not understand the verb in this sentence, "reads" is a much more likely response than "owns," making the sentence with "reads" more semantically predictable. Sentences that are more predictable result in higher intelligibility scores than those with less predictability (Boothroyd & Nittrouer, 1988; Duffy & Giolas, 1974; Garcia & Cannito, 1996). Studies have found higher intelligibility when there is cohesion between sentences (meaning the sentences are related to each other) than when sentences are unrelated (Drager & Reichle, 2001; Hustad & Beukelman, 2002). When you plan your assessment, consider syntactic and semantic predictability, as well as cohesion of the sentences you choose and, if comparing, be sure to use similar levels.

Presentation Mode of Message

When planning intelligibility measures, SLPs should consider how the message will be presented to listeners, which we will describe as presentation mode. As a practical matter, most intelligibility measures will take place using recorded stimuli. Instructions in the Frenchay Dysarthria Test—Second Edition (Enderby & Palmer, 2008) state that transcription can be completed online (as the client is speaking) by the clinician or can be recorded for later transcription. Recording your client's production of the message will allow you to separate the speaker and listener tasks. If you are using an audio or audio/video recorder, it is important to carefully control the environment where the speaker is recorded.

Give careful consideration to the type of recording and whether you use audio or video recording during intelligibility measures. Details of standardized assessments for intelligibility, listed in Table 4–1 show that most measures involve the use of audio-only stimuli. Studies comparing audio-only and auditory-visual intelligibility measures across speakers have shown us that including visual information can influence intelligibility scores in speakers with various communication disorders. Studies examining visual influence in dysarthria have included speakers with Parkinson's disease (Keintz et al., 2007), cerebral palsy (Hustad & Cahill, 2003; Hunter et al., 1991) and multiple dysarthria types resulting from various neurogenic conditions (Barkmeier, 1988). While most of these studies showed some speakers had higher intelligibility scores in auditory-visual conditions, the findings are definitely inconsistent and affected by severity of dysarthria, presentation mode (if auditory-only was presented first or second to listeners), and other complicating factors. Intelligibility in alaryngeal speakers was found to improve when visual information is included (Evitts et al., 2009) but again, this gain would probably depend on many other factors.

A solid take-home point from these studies is that inclusion of visual information can influence intelligibility scores (for better or for worse), and you should not compare measures with different presentation modes. Because the results could vary on a case-by-case basis, SLPs should consider the visual aspects of the individual they are evaluating. It is possible that speakers with distracting or reduced facial movements may actually have a negative impact on their intelligibility if listeners see their face. But, in other cases, we can assume that listeners will take advantage of the extra information from facial movements. Whereas listeners can understand non-disordered speech without having visual information, speakers with reduced intelligibility may be better understood with visual information provided. We want to be sure we are consistent in pretreatment and posttreatment measures in regard to procedures using facemasks. If you are recording a speaker, ensure that the microphone is not touching their face and after you assist the speaker with putting on the microphone, step away and ask them to remove their mask (Magee et al., 2020). Following these procedures will help you with consistent measures of both auditory and visual information.

Factors Related to Listeners

Listeners in intelligibility measures are asked to complete a very different task than what they do as communicators in real-life situations. In functional communication, the listener will perceive the speaker's message, respond, and interact. During a structured assessment, the listener performs a one-sided task with no feedback or method to repair any breakdowns in communication. According to McHenry (2011), a more realistic assessment will result in more subjectivity in scoring. This subjectivity can contribute to variability among listeners, which can lead to less reliable results of an intelligibility assessment.

Individual Listener Variability

When we obtain intelligibility measures using different listeners, there are many variables that occur between individuals. Different listeners do not have the same internal standards for what they consider to be a normal voice (Muñoz et al., 2002). Investigations have found variability between listeners in studies of voice quality (Kempster et al., 2009; Kreiman et al., 2007) and nasality (Watterson et al., 2007). Eadie and colleagues (2010) found that a listener's musical background affected how listeners rated dysphonia. Training improves reliability in some listeners (Eadie & Baylor, 2006), which could be helpful as a management strategy but does not help us protect against variability during assessment. On a functional note, we may have to accept variability between listeners during assessment, but other factors that are in our control can be minimized and will be discussed next.

Listener Task

The listener task varies depending on the type of intelligibility measure you are using. Table 4.1 provides information on listener tasks for various assessment choices. Both the SIT (Yorkston et al., 2007) and MWIT (Kent et al., 1989) are set up to allow the listener to choose between a set limit (4–6) choices like a multiple-choice test for single words. The AIDS (Yorkston & Beukelman, 1984) has a transcription or forced choice option. Higher scores are noted on word tests where the listener has the choices, as opposed to wide-open transcription tasks (McHenry, 2011). Clinicians using transcription of sentences may gain useful information about longer, more functional utterances. This method could result in lower intelligibility scores related to the speaker's challenge with intelligibility on longer utterances as well as the listener's ability to remember and transcribe the longer utterance (McHenry, 2011). Given the number of variables that affect the listener's task, there is not a simple answer for what is best. Consider the needs of your client and abilities of your listeners. It is important to be consistent if you are measuring the same client over time as changes in listener task may impact the outcome.

Experience

Experienced listeners are those who may be used to hearing disordered speakers or even specific types of disordered speech, like that produced by individuals with Parkinson's disease. It is common for research studies that need larger numbers of listeners to recruit from university students, sometimes, even students from communication sciences and disorders programs. This means many of the listeners are younger and mostly female. You could ask questions to exclude listeners who may have experience in working with clients with similar disorders or even family members. Several investigations comparing experienced SLP transcription versus inexperienced individuals found that experience resulted in higher intelligibility scores in speakers with dysarthria (Barkmeier, 1988) and alaryngeal speech (Doyle et al., 1988; Finizia et al., 1998). Several other studies did not find differences between experienced SLPs and other listeners considered to be inexperienced (Hunter et al., 1991; Keintz et al., 2007). There may be cases where having another SLP as a listener might be helpful if professional insight into what is impacting intelligibility is needed. If your goal is to learn how real-world listeners will understand your client, using listeners who are not experienced with disordered speech in general, or their specific disorder characteristics, is the best way to go.

Familiarity With Speaker

To differentiate from experience, familiarity with the speaker refers to listeners who have previously heard and perhaps learned speech patterns of your client. Research supports that exposure to speakers and/or messages will provide listeners with an advantage (Borrie et al., 2012a, 2012b; D'Innocenzo et al., 2006; Liss et al., 2002; Utianski et al., 2011;). When we are planning management, we can use this familiarity positively to improve intelligibility (see Chapter 7). In the case of assessment, however, we want to control for these factors.

Consider what you want to learn from the assessment. If you want to know how family or close friends communicate with your client, using them as listeners will provide that information. We just want to remember that these familiar listeners will have more knowledge about what their family members like to talk about, what they think about topics, and they will be familiar with the way the client speaks. If you have interest in knowing how unfamiliar listeners, such as restaurant servers, telemarketers, or bank tellers, understand your client, you will want to select listeners who are not familiar with your client. Unfamiliar listeners may also be affected by how motivated they are to successfully communicate and how much attention they will put into the process (Tjaden & Liss, 1995).

Familiarity With Message

Regarding assessment, we want to consider what the listener is transcribing. Imagine if we had the speaker recite the pledge of allegiance and then asked a listener to transcribe it. They would have a very predictable message to decipher, and we wouldn't expect there to be many errors. Studies that have looked at listener familiarity with the message have shown us that intelligibility is increased when the message is something listeners have heard previously (Beukelman & Yorkston, 1980; Tjaden & Liss, 1995; Yorkston & Beukelman, 1978). Improved scores following exposure to speakers or stimuli can work to our advantage in some management situations. But, for assessment, we want to use listeners and the message from the speakers consistently. If you are measuring intelligibility frequently, change listeners to avoid them becoming familiar with the speaker. Changing sentence lists or stimuli may also help avoid listeners learning the message. If you use a different listener, you will avoid previous exposure to the message as well. It is pretty obvious that transcribing a speech sample that you recorded yourself will result in several issues discussed in this section. You should find other listeners and consider the influence of the factors discussed here to have the most functional measures of intelligibility for your clients.

Age

Listener age is another factor that can influence intelligibility scores. Studies that have examined age as a listener factor have not consistently grouped ages into "older" and "younger" categories. Generally, the younger group ranged from between the ages 18 to 30, and older groups fell between the ages 65 to 80, or had no cutoff after 80 years of age. Studies were conducted with speakers who exihibited reduced intelligibility related to dysarthria, and consistently, older listeners did not perform as well on listening tasks related to intelligibility (Dagenais et al., 2011; Jones et al., 2004; McAuliffe et al., 2017). Several factors could influence the abilities of older listeners on these types of tasks, including hearing ability, attention, and cognitive issues. It would be easy to dismiss older listeners in our assessments and just use younger individuals for listening tasks. This may not be at all representative of who our client's communicative partners are. It is critical to consider your listeners and recruit people who are similar to those your client will communicate with. You may want to perform a simple hearing screening on potential listeners to ensure that hearing loss isn't affecting the results. We will revisit this topic in Chapter 7 when we discuss what your client's communicative partners can do to improve their ability to hear and understand.

Factors Related to the Communicative Environment

When you are assessing intelligibility, the communicative environment will need to be considered more than one time. Initially, you will need to plan for factors related to recording the speaker. A second consideration involves the environment where the listener completed their task. As we've mentioned before, if you measure a client's intelligibility under one set of conditions and then complete a posttreatment measure, your communication environment should be consistent for both speaker and listener tasks to control for influence of the environment.

Recording Equipment

For a complete discussion of the equipment that is best used to record your client, see Chapter 3. Using high-quality speech samples that are recorded consistently using the same equipment and mouth to microphone distance will ensure comparable recordings. Keeping careful notes on each client's recording will ensure you know exactly how to proceed on any subsequent recordings after the initial assessment.

Auditory-Only Versus Auditory-Visual Presentation Mode

As discussed earlier in this chapter, researchers have found that visual information influences intelligibility scores in speakers with dysarthria (Barkmeier, 1988; Hunter et al., 1991; Hustad & Cahill, 2003; Keintz et al., 2007) and those using alaryngeal speech (Evitts et al., 2009). Factors such as speaker severity and presentation order (whether the listeners heard auditory-only or auditory-visual first) influenced the results of these studies. For the most part, they found higher intelligibility scores when listeners had access to both auditory and visual information. Clinicians should consider this factor and, at the least, not compare recordings, including visual information with those that contain auditory samples only.

Listening Conditions

You want to have some control over the conditions where your listener is transcribing or rating the speech sample. Mainly so that when you want to reevaluate your client's intelligibility, you can measure it the same way you obtained their pretreatment level. If your first measure involved a listener in a noisy environment, but your second listening session was completed in a soundproof booth, you would expect different results based only on that fact, but your client's intelligibility would most likely appear to have improved. Options for listening environments can vary greatly. In many research studies, a soundproof booth is used to allow the most control of the environment. However, most clinicians would not have easy access to a booth and if you think about it, that type of environment is not a realistic comparison to anyone's communication environment. Background noise added using computer programs has been shown to decrease intelligibility in speakers with dysphonia more than in speakers with non-disordered voices (Ishikawa et al., 2017). Similar decreased intelligibility in background noise has been noted in speakers with dysarthria as well (Lee et al., 2011; Dykstra et al., 2012; Yoho & Borrie, 2018). Having listeners complete transcription in quiet, controlled environments, even with noise added, allows researchers to determine the impact of different factors. However, for clinical practice, consider the client's needs and situation. There is no clear-cut answer to how best to control the communicative environment. Knowing that your client's intelligibility could be inflated in perfect listening conditions is a good start. If you know the listening environment is consistent between measures, at least that one factor is under your control.

ASSESSMENT OF COMPREHENSIBILITY, EFFICIENCY, AND NATURALNESS

There are many factors to control or keep constant across measures if we want to have accurate measures of intelligibility. When we add this control, we are basically removing contextual information that would normally be available to listeners in everyday conversations. If we want to have a useful measure of communicative effectiveness, including these functional cues, we can create measures where the listener has access to more than just speech sounds. Comprehensibility is a type of intelligibility, but we are adding consideration of other factors, including gestures, context, and semantic cues for listeners to use in decoding the message. Written cues from the speaker or an alphabet board could also be included. By this definition, if you want to assess comprehensibility by including these factors, you will consider the speaker, message, listener, and other environmental factors. If your assessment includes visual cues of any type (e.g., speaker's facial cues/movements, gestures, written cues), use audio/visual recordings to allow the listener to use this information. We have not developed standardized assessment tests to measure comprehensibility. Determining which cues and information to provide can be completed on a patient-specific basis. For instance, if you want to know if using gestures would be a good target for treatment, you can assess differences when listeners see the gestures and when they do not. You can compare measures of a client providing semantic cues to when the cues are not available to the listener. For example, you could have the client read a list of ice cream flavors and determine if listeners understand more if they are told that the client will name flavors of ice cream. This will help you determine if teaching the client to present these types of cues will improve communication effectiveness.

You may also want to include measures that assess listener comprehension rather than the ability to transcribe utterances. Comprehension extends the concept of intelligibility as it can measure the listener's ability to summarize the speaker's message (Higginbotham et al., 1994), or respond to questions about the message (Hustad & Beukelman, 2002). For a comprehension task, reading passages could be used along with questions for the listener to answer. Hustad (2008) used two types of questions in a study comparing intelligibility and comprehension measures. In her methods, inferential questions were developed in which the answer could be inferred but was not directly stated in the passage. Factual questions were developed where the answers were directly in what was read in the passage. The results showed that including measures of both intelligibility and comprehension can lead to an effective management plan. Duffy (2019) suggests we consider the differences between intelligibility and comprehensibility and the impact of efficiency on both in assessing clients. He mentions that estimates of a speaker's intelligibility and efficiency provide a measure of how impaired the speech is. And estimates of comprehensibility and efficiency measure the impact of the speech disorder on the speaker's ability to participate in activities that involve communication. Swigert (2010) suggests observation of cues and strategies clients may be implementing during conversation. She advises clinicians to describe how cues are used, what listeners do to facilitate communication, and whether the cues appear to improve communication.

Efficiency refers to how quickly the speaker shares information and has a relationship with both intelligibility and comprehensibility. Measures of efficiency can provide you with useful information about the listener's perception of how normal the speech sounds. A disordered speaker may have fairly high intelligibility, but a low level of efficiency because of a very slow rate of speech. A speaker can have very reduced intelligibility, because of a more severe disorder where slowing rate doesn't change how much listeners understand. This person may use gestures or written cues to help listeners which will improve comprehensibility but decrease efficiency. The Perceptual Dysarthria Evaluation (PDE; Swigert, 2010) is an excellent resource for subjective descriptions and considerations of comprehensibility and efficiency. The Assessment of Intelligibility of Dysarthric Speech (AIDS; Yorkston & Beukelman, 1984) and Sentence Intelligibilty Test (SIT; Yorkston et al., 2007) contain measures of rate and efficiency.

Speech naturalness refers to the overall adequacy of prosody (Duffy, 2019). Reduced naturalness is often associated with unnatural speaking rate, inappropriate pauses or changes in rhythm, intonation, or timing that is expected by listeners (Lowit et al., 2022). According to Lowit and colleagues (2022), rather than applying a percentage or scale judgment, clinicians usually state whether prosody is affected. Chapter 3 contains discussion of assessment procedures related to prosody. As prosody can affect both intelligibility and naturalness, it is important to assess this area to determine how improved prosody may impact overall communication effectiveness (Lowit et al., 2022).

INTELLIGIBILITY MEASURES RELATED TO VOICE DISORDERS AND HEAD AND NECK CANCER

It is important to note that most of the research on intelligibility and the related concepts discussed in this chapter have examined clients with dysarthria. Studies of intelligibility related to voice disorders are fairly recent, but show that reduced intelligibility can occur in individuals with voice disorders who have intact articulation (Evitts et al., 2016; Ma et al., 2021; Porcaro et al., 2020). Specific tests and measures for intelligibility in clients with voice disorders have not yet been created, but these studies have pointed out the need to consider intelligibility factors. Ishikawa and colleagues (2020) compared measures of intelligibility in individuals with dysphonia and determined that rating scale and transcription task were highly correlated, which tells us that rating scales may be a useful, time-saving method of measuring intelligibility with some clients.

Assessment in clients with H&N cancer can also be a challenge, in that specific intelligibility tests have not yet been designed. Related to clients who have undergone laryngectomy, Doyle (2019b) points out that no matter which type of alaryngeal speech is used, it will be identified as abnormal by listeners. But abnormal does not always mean unintelligible, and it is useful to have a measure of the client's intelligibility. Voice quality and resonance are important factors in this population and the impact on intelligibility will vary from client to client. For these reasons, it is critical to consider the subsystem assessment (See Chapter 3) in addition to controlled measures of intelligibility for a complete picture. Constantinescu and Rieger (2019) suggest use of the Frenchay Dysarthria Assessment-2nd edition (FDA-2), London Speech Evaluation (LSE), and SIT (see Tables 3–1, 3–4, and 4–1) in evaluation of oral and oropharyngeal cancer. Eadie (2019) reminds us that documentation of participation restrictions and impact on social functioning is important for clients with H&N cancer. Several options for these types of measures have been developed for other populations but may be useful in some cases (Table 3–5). For clinicians working with the H&N cancer population, Doyle's book, Clinical Care and

Rehabilitation in Head and Neck Cancer (2019a) is an excellent resource for evaluation considerations.

USE OF TECHNOLOGY IN INTELLIGIBILITY ASSESSMENT

Previous studies and enhanced technology are leading to some interesting possibilities for future intelligibility measures. The Communication Related Parameters for Speech Disorders (KommPaS; Lehner & Ziegler, 2021) is a web-based assessment currently available only in German. This word intelligibility test allows selection from over 12,000 words. Speakers with dysarthria are recorded using KommPaS reading these words in carrier sentences that are neutral in syntax and semantics. Listeners unfamiliar with the speakers are recruited by crowdsourcing through (enlisting the services of people on the Internet) and they complete a word transcription task. A grand profile containing measures of intelligibility, naturalness, efficiency, and perceived listener effort will be available when using KommPaS. As of 2021, reliability, validity, and feasibility studies are needed but there is strong potential in using this type of assessment.

Borrie and colleagues (2019) have created a software tool for scoring intelligibility called Autoscore. This tool is open source, so it is available at no cost and can be modified and redistributed. This software scores what a listener has already transcribed so you will need to have that step completed if you want to use it. You can access Autoscore at http://autoscore .usu.edu/ to use in your clinical practice. When you log in to this site, they will ask you first to choose a set of rules that will be used for transcription of the speech sample. An example of a rule you can set is whether to count "assumed" as a correct response for "assume" or not. After you select the sets of rules you want to apply, you will upload a document containing the target words/phrases as well as what the listener transcribed. After Autoscore has analyzed what you submitted, you will see an interactive table on the screen that gives you scoring information. Other investigations have used speech recognition software to examine phoneme and word boundaries (Jiao et al., 2019) and future studies related to these methods may produce clinical tools to help us automate the process of intelligibility measurement.

Haley (2011) developed a one-word intelligibility test that utilizes computer software that provides a model for the speaker and records the message. A listener's transcriptions are then scored by the software, which gives you an intelligibility score at word level. This software, known as the Chapel Hill Multilingual Intelligibility Test, has been developed for use with at least ten languages and is available free of cost (see Table 4–1). If you are technologically savvy, some of these options that allow for electronic assistance may be helpful.

SUMMARY

Measures of intelligibility can provide relevant information at baseline to determine management targets, as well as indications of effects of treatment. Many SLPs indicate they do not use intelligibility measures when evaluating adult clients due to lack of availability of formal measures or lack of knowledge of procedures. Investigations of intelligibility measurement have shown that many factors related to the speaker and message can influence scores. Factors related to the speaker include severity of the disorder and rate of speech. The speaker's message can be affected by multiple factors, including type of message (words versus sentences), the predictability of the message, and whether visual information is available to the listeners. Listener-related factors can include age, experience with a speaker group, experience with the speaker or message, and the task used. The communication environment can be influenced by choices in how the speaker is recorded and how the listener is presented with the recording. Following consistent procedures, with attention paid to these factors, will provide more accurate measures that allow for comparison of results over time. A checklist is provided in Appendix 4–3 to remind you of factors to consider during assessment.

Case Study

Dysarthria Case: Jack's SLP, Christy, took a holistic approach to assessment of his intelligibility by gaining information from many potential communicative partners and environments. Christy administered the Sentence Intelligibility Test (SIT; Yorkston et al., 2007) by audio recording of Jack reading the sentences in a sound-attenuated room. She knew this was an optimal setting with no background noise, but wanted this measure as a baseline where environmental noise was eliminated as an influence on later scores. With Jack's permission, Christy asked a colleague who works in the billing department of her hospital to listen to the sentences and indicate on the computer what he heard in a quiet room. This listener was chosen because he did not know Jack, which eliminated speaker familiarity and none of Jack's information was provided to the listener. Her colleague also did not have extensive experience with individuals with dysarthria. Results of the SIT indicated 74% intelligibility with mildly slower than normal rate of speech.

Christy had observed some unexpected oral movements during conversation with Jack, so she planned an informal intelligibility assessment using both audio and visual information. She used sets 2 and 4 from Medical Research Council (MRC) Institute of Hearing Research (MacLeod & Summerfield, 1990) audio-visual sentence lists (See Appendix 4–1), which allowed her to have 30 sentences that were unpredictable and equalized for the visual information provided. She recorded Jack using both video and audio recorders and asked two individuals to transcribe what they heard, including a friend from his class and one of his professors. These individuals had some level of familiarity with Jack's speech, but they also represented functional listeners in his daily life. Christy asked the listeners to transcribe in an empty classroom on campus where there was minimal noise in the room itself, but muffled noise from the hallway. She knew this was not an ideal listening environment, but perhaps one that more accurately reflected Jack's typical communication situation. Results of this informal assessment revealed that Jack's friend understood 79% of his words in sentences and his professor understood 73%. Christy took careful notes during these intelligibility assessments because she knew that in order to compare scores, she will need to replicate the same conditions when she takes posttreatment measures.

Case Study

Voice Disorders Case: Thomas wanted to measure the impact of Beth's voice quality on intelligibility. Although the teletherapy environment created challenges for him, his skills with intelligibility assessment and technology allowed him to complete this evaluation task. His goal was to create tasks that he could replicate and provide functional information to help formulate goals with Beth. He instructed her to read sentences from the Sentence Intelligibility Test (SIT; Yorkston et al., 2007) while he recorded both audio and video channels using his clinic's encrypted recording system. To gain information on how unfamiliar listeners understood her speech, Thomas received written permission from Beth to have a colleague who is a physical therapist in his facility transcribe the sentences in a quiet room. Thomas' colleague understood 86% of the words in Beth's sentences through this manner of transcription. The colleague reported that he felt her soft speech was difficult to understand and that he felt he relied on her mouth and lip movements to help determine what some of the words were. To learn about Beth's intelligibility with family members, Thomas asked her daughter to transcribe the same sentences from the SIT (Yorkston et al., 2007) at home during a time of day when everyone was home. She sat in a room near the family but not in the same room. She placed the sound pressure level (SPL) meter 12 inches from herself at the table and noted the reading of 52 dB SLP. Beth's daughter was able to understand 92% of her utterances in this typical home listening environment.

REFERENCES

Barkmeier, J. M. (1988). *Intelligibility of dysarthric speakers: Audio-only and audio-visual presentations.* [Master's thesis, University of Iowa]. Iowa Research Online.https://iro.uiowa.edu/esploro/outputs/graduate/998377 6831702771

Barreto, S. S., & Ortiz, K. Z. (2020). Speech intelligibility in dysarthrias: Influence of utterance length. *Folia Phoniatrica et Logopaedica, 72*(3), 202–210. https://doi.org/10.1159/000497178

Bench, J., Kowal, A., & Bamford, J. (1979). The BKB (Bamford-Kowal-Bench) sentence lists for partially-hearing children. *British Journal of Audiology, 13*(3), 108–112. https://doi.org/10.3109/03005367909078884

Beukelman, D. R., & Yorkston, K. M. (1980). Influence of passage familiarity on intelligibility estimates of dysarthric speech. *Journal of Communication Disorders, 13*(1), 33–41. https://doi.org/10.1016/0021-9924(80)90019-2

Boothroyd, A., & Nittrouer, S. (1988). Mathematical treatment of context effects in phoneme and word recognition. *The Journal of the Acoustical Society of America, 84*(1), 101–114. https://doi.org/10.1121/1.396976

Borrie, S. A., Barrett, T. S., & Yoho, S. E. (2019). Autoscore: An open-source automated tool for scoring listener perception of speech. *The Journal of the Acoustical Society of America, 145*(1), 392–399. https://doi.org/10 .1121/1.5087276

Borrie, S. A., McAuliffe, M. J., & Liss, J. M. (2012a). Perceptual learning of dysarthric speech: A review of experimental studies. *Journal of Speech, Language, and Hearing Research, 55*(1), 290–305. https://doi.org/10 .1044/1092-4388(2011/10-0349)

Borrie, S. A., McAuliffe, M. J., Liss, J. M., O'Beirne, G. A., & Anderson, T. J. (2012b). A follow-up investigation into the mechanisms that underlie improved recognition of dysarthric speech. *The Journal of the Acoustical Society of America, 132*(2), EL102–EL108. https://doi.org/10.1121/1 .4736952

Carter, C., Yorkston, K., Strand, E., & Hammen, V. (1996). Effects of semantic and syntactic context on actual and estimated sentence intelligibility of dysarthric speakers. In D. Robin, K. Yorkston, & D. Beukelman (Eds.), *Disorders of motor speech: Assessment, treatment, and clinical characterization* (pp. 67–87). Paul H. Brookes.

Collis, J., & Bloch, S. (2012). Survey of UK speech and language therapists' assessment and treatment practices for people with progressive dysarthria. *International Journal of Language & Communication Disorders, 47*(6), 725–737. https://doi.org/10.1111/j.1460-6984.2012.00183.x

Constantinescu, G., & Rieger, J. M. (2019). Speech deficits associated with oral and oropharyngeal carcinomas. In P. C. Doyle (Ed.), *Clinical care and rehabilitation in head and neck cancer.* (pp. 265–279). Springer. https:// doi.org/10.1007/978-3-030-04702-3_16

Dagenais, P. A., Adlington, L. M., & Evans, K. J. (2011). Intelligibility, comprehensibility, and acceptability of dysarthric speech by older and younger listeners. *Journal of Medical Speech-Language Pathology, 19*(4), 37–48.

D'Innocenzo, J., Tjaden, K., & Greenman, G. (2006) Intelligibility in dysarthria: Effects of listener familiarity and speaking condition. *Clinical Linguistics & Phonetics, 20*(9), 659–675. https://doi.org/10.1080/026992005 00224272

Dolgova, Y., & Haley, K. L. (2011). *Chapel Hill Multilingual Intelligibility Test, Russian Version*. Center for Aphasia and Related Disorders. https://www .med.unc.edu/ahs/sphs/card/wp-content/uploads/sites/486/2018/02/Rus sian.pdf

Doyle, P. C. (Ed.). (2019a). *Clinical care and rehabilitation in head and neck cancer*. Springer. https://doi.org/10.1007/978-3-030-04702-3

Doyle, P. C. (2019b). Documenting voice and speech outcomes in alaryngeal speakers. In P. C. Doyle (Ed.), *Clinical care and rehabilitation in head and neck cancer* (pp. 281–297). Springer. https://doi.org/10.1007/978 -3-030-04702-3_17

Doyle, P. C., Danhauer, J. L., & Reed, C. G. (1988). Listeners' perceptions of consonants produced by esophageal and tracheosophageal talkers. *Journal of Speech and Hearing Disorders, 53*(4), 400–407. https://doi.org/10.1044 /jshd.5304.400

Drager, K. D., & Reichle, J. E. (2001). Effects of discourse context on the intelligibility of synthesized speech for young adult and older adult listeners: Applications for AAC. *Journal of Speech, Language, and Hearing Research, 44*(5), 1052–1057. https://doi.org/10.1044/1092-4388(2001/083)

Duffy, J. R. (2019). *Motor speech disorders: Substrates, differential diagnosis, and management* (4th ed.). Elsevier.

Duffy, J. R., & Giolas, T. G. (1974). Sentence intelligibility as a function of key word selection. *Journal of Speech and Hearing Research, 17*(4), 631–637. https://doi.org/10.1044/jshr.1704.631

Dykstra, A. D., Adams, S. G., & Jog, M. (2012). The effect of background noise on the speech intensity of individuals with hypophonia associated with Parkinson's disease. *Journal of Medical Speech-Language Pathology, 20*(3), 19–30.

Eadie T. L. (2019). Communicative participation after head and neck cancer. In P. C. Doyle (Ed.), *Clinical care and rehabilitation in head and neck cancer* (pp. 483–497). Springer. https://doi.org/10.1007/978-3-030-04702-3_29

Eadie, T. L., & Baylor, C. R. (2006). The effect of perceptual training on inexperienced listeners' judgments of dysphonic voice. *Journal of Voice, 20*(4), 527–544. https://doi.org/10.1016/j.jvoice.2005.08.007

Eadie, T. L., Van Boven, L., Stubbs, K., & Giannini, E. (2010). The effect of musical background on judgments of dysphonia. *Journal of Voice, 24*(1), 93–101. https://doi.org/10.1016/j.jvoice.2008.04.008

Enderby, P., & Palmer, R. (2008). *Frenchay Dysarthria Assessment-Second Edition (FDA-2): Manual*. Pro-Ed.

Evitts, P. M., Starmer, H., Teets, K., Montgomery, C., Calhoun, L., Schulze, A., . . . Adams, L. (2016). The impact of dysphonic voices on healthy listeners: Listener reaction times, speech intelligibility, and listener comprehension. *American Journal of Speech-Language Pathology*, *25*(4), 561–575. https://doi.org/10.1044/2016_AJSLP-14-0183

Evitts, P. M., Van Dine, A., & Holler, A. (2009). Effects of audio-visual information and mode of speech on listener perceptions of alaryngeal speakers. *International Journal of Speech-Language Pathology*, *11*(6), 450–460. https://doi.org/10.3109/17549500903003078

Fairbanks, G. (1960). *Voice and articulation drillbook* (2nd ed.). Harper & Row.

Finizia, C., Lindström, J., & Dotevall, H. (1998). Intelligibility and perceptual ratings after treatment for laryngeal cancer: Laryngectomy vs. radiotherapy. *Laryngoscope*, *108*(1), 138–143. https://doi.org/10.1097/00005537-199801000-00027

Fischer, L., & Haley, K. L. (2014). *Chapel Hill Multilingual Intelligibility Test, Spanish Version (bisyllabic words)*. Center for Aphasia and Related Disorders. https://www.med.unc.edu/ahs/sphs/card/wp-content/uploads/sites/486/2018/02/Spanish.pdf

Fontan, L., Tardieu, J., Gaillard, P., Woisard, V., & Ruiz, R. (2015). Relationship between speech intelligibility and speech comprehension in babble noise. *Journal of Speech, Language, and Hearing Research*, *58*(3), 977–986. https://doi.org/10.1044/2015_JSLHR-H-13-0335

Gammelgaard, E., & Haley, K. L. (2016). *Chapel Hill Multilingual Intelligibility Test, Danish Version (monosyllabic words)*. Center for Aphasia and Related Disorders. https://www.med.unc.edu/ahs/sphs/card/wp-content/uploads/sites/486/2018/02/Danish.pdf

Garcia, J. M., & Cannito, M. P. (1996). Influence of verbal and nonverbal contexts on the sentence intelligibility of a speaker with dysarthria. *Journal of Speech, Language, and Hearing Research*, *39*(4), 750–760. https://doi.org/10.1044/jshr.3904.750

Gery, A., & Haley, K. L. (2011). *Chapel Hill Multilingual Intelligibility Test, Swedish Version (monosyllabic words)*. Center for Aphasia and Related Disorders. https://www.med.unc.edu/ahs/sphs/card/wp-content/uploads/sites/486/2018/02/Swedish.pdf

Gurevich, N., & Scamihorn, S. L. (2017). Speech-language pathologists' use of intelligibility measures in adults with dysarthria. *American Journal of Speech-Language Pathology*, *26*(3), 873–892. https://doi.org/10.1044/2017_ajslp-16-0112

Haley, K. L. (2011). *Chapel Hill Multilingual Intelligibility Test, English Version (monosyllabic words)*. Center for Aphasia and Related Disorders. https://www.med.unc.edu/ahs/sphs/card/wp-content/uploads/sites/486/2018/02/English.pdf

Hammen, V. L., Yorkston, K. M., & Minifie, F. D. (1994). Effects of temporal alterations on speech intelligibility in parkinsonian dysarthria. *Journal of Speech, Language, and Hearing Research*, *37*(2), 244–253. https://doi.org/10.1044/jshr.3702.244

Higginbotham, D. J., Drazek, A., Kowarsky, K., Scally, C., & Segal, E. (1994). Discourse comprehension of synthetic speech delivered at normal and slow presentation rates. *Augmentative and Alternative Communication, 10*(3), 191–202. https://doi.org/10.1080/07434619412331276900

Hunter, L., Pring, T., & Martin, S. (1991). The use of strategies to increase speech intelligibility in cerebral palsy: An experimental evaluation. *International Journal of Language & Communication Disorders, 26*(2), 163–174. https://doi.org/10.3109/13682829109012001

Hustad, K. C. (2006). A closer look at transcription intelligibility for speakers with dysarthria: Evaluation of scoring paradigms and linguistic errors made by listeners. *American Journal of Speech Language Pathology, 15*(3), 268–277. https://doi.org/10.1044/1058-0360(2006/025)

Hustad, K. C. (2007). Effects of speech stimuli and dysarthria severity on intelligibility scores and listener confidence ratings for speakers with cerebral palsy. *Folia Phoniatrica et Logopaedica, 59*(6), 306–317. https://doi.org/10.1159/000108337

Hustad, K. C. (2008). The relationship between listener comprehension and intelligibility scores for speakers with dysarthria. *Journal of Speech, Language, and Hearing Research, 51*(3), 562–573. https://doi.org/10.1044/1092-4388(2008/040)

Hustad, K. C., & Beukelman, D. R. (2002). Listener comprehension of severely dysarthric speech: Effects of linguistic cues and stimulus cohesion. *Journal of Speech, Language, and Hearing Research, 45*(3), 545–558. https://doi.org/10.1044/1092-4388(2002/043)

Hustad, K. C., & Cahill, M. A. (2003). Effects of presentation mode and repeated familiarization on intelligibility of dysarthric speech. *American Journal of Speech-Language Pathology, 12*(2), 198–208. https://doi.org/10.1044/1058-0360(2003/066)

Hustad, K. C., & Weismer, G. (2007). A continuum of interventions for individuals with dysarthria: Compensatory and rehabilitative treatment approaches. In G. Weismer (Ed.), *Motor speech disorders: Essays for Ray Kent* (pp. 261–303). Plural Publishing.

Ishikawa, K., Boyce, S., Kelchner, L., Powell, M. G., Schieve, H., de Alarcon, A., & Khosla, S. (2017). The effect of background noise on intelligibility of dysphonic speech. *Journal of Speech, Language, and Hearing Research, 60*(7), 1919–1929. https://doi.org/10.1044/2017_JSLHR-S-16-0012

Ishikawa, K., Webster, J., & Ketring, C. (2020). Agreement between transcription- and rating-based intelligibility measurements for evaluation of dysphonic speech in noise. *Clinical Linguistics & Phonetics*, 1–13. https://doi.org/10.1080/02699206.2020.1852602

Jiao, Y., LaCross, A., Berisha, V., & Liss, J. (2019). Objective intelligibility assessment by automated segmental and suprasegmental listening error analysis. *Journal of Speech, Language, and Hearing Research, 62*(9), 3359–3366. https://doi.org/10.1044/2019_jslhr-s-19-0119

Jones, W., Mathy, P., Azuma, T., & Liss, J. M. (2004). The effect of aging and synthetic topic cues on the intelligibility of dysarthric speech. *Augmentative and Alternative Communication, 20*(1), 22–29. https://doi.org/10.1080/07 434610310001615981

Jozefowicz, S., & Haley, K. L. (2011). *Chapel Hill Multilingual Intelligibility Test, French Version (monosyllabic words).* Center for Aphasia and Related Disorders. https://www.med.unc.edu/ahs/sphs/card/wp-content/uploads /sites/486/2018/02/French.pdf

Keintz, C. K., Bunton, K., & Hoit, J. D. (2007). Influence of visual information on the intelligibility of dysarthric speech. *American Journal of Speech-Language Pathology, 16*(3), 222–234. https://doi.org/10.1044/1058-0360(2007/027)

Kempster, G. B., Gerratt, B. R., Verdolini Abbott, K., Barkmeier-Kraemer, J., & Hillman, R. E. (2009). Consensus auditory-perceptual evaluation of voice: Development of a standardized clinical protocol. *American Journal of Speech-Language Pathology, 18*(2), 124–132.

Kent, R. D., Weismer, G., Kent, J. F., & Rosenbek, J. C. (1989). Toward phonetic intelligibility testing in dysarthria. *Journal of Speech and Hearing Disorders, 54*(4), 482–499. https://doi.org/10.1044/jshd.5404.482

King, J. M., Watson, M., & Lof, G. L. (2012). Practice patterns of speech-language pathologists assessing intelligibility of dysarthric speech. *Journal of Medical Speech-Language Pathology, 20*(1), 1–16.

Klasner, E. R., & Yorkston, K. M. (2005). Speech intelligibility in ALS and HD dysarthria: The everyday listener's perspective. *Journal of Medical Speech-Language Pathology, 13*(2), 127–139.

Kreiman, J., Gerratt, B. R., & Ito, M. (2007). When and why listeners disagree in voice quality assessment tasks. *The Journal of the Acoustical Society of America, 122*(4), 2354–2364. https://doi.org/10.1121/1.2770547

Lee, Y., Sim, H. S., & Sung, J. E. (2011). Effects of the types of noise and signal-to-noise ratios on speech intelligibility in dysarthria. *Phonetics and Speech Sciences, 3*(4), 117–124.

Lehner, K., & Ziegler, W. (2021). The impact of lexical and articulatory factors in the automatic selection of test materials for a web-based assessment of intelligibility in dysarthria. *Journal of Speech, Language, and Hearing Research, 64*(6S), 2196–2212. https://doi.org/10.1044/2020_JSLHR-20-00267

Liss, J. M., Spitzer, S. M., Caviness, J. N., Adler, C., & Edwards, B. W. (2000). Lexical boundary error analysis in hypokinetic and ataxic dysarthria. *The Journal of the Acoustical Society of America, 107*(6), 3415–3424. https://doi.org/10.1121/1.429412

Liss, J. M., Spitzer, S. M., Caviness, J. N., & Adler, C. (2002). The effects of familiarization on intelligibility and lexical segmentation in hypokinetic and ataxic dysarthria. *The Journal of Acoustical Society of America, 112*(6), 3022–3030. https://doi.org/10.1121/1.1515793

Lowit, A., & Kent, R. D. (2011). *Assessment of motor speech disorders.* Plural Publishing.

Lowit, A., Kent, R. D., & Kuschmann, A. (2022). Management of dysarthria. In I. Papathanasiou & P. Coppens (Eds.), *Aphasia and related neurogenic communication disorders* (3rd ed., pp. 641–671). Jones & Bartlett Learning.

Ma, E. P., Tse, M. M., Momenian, M., Pu, D., & Chen, F. F. (2021). The effects of dysphonic voice on speech intelligibility in Cantonese-speaking adults. *Journal of Speech, Language, and Hearing Research*, *64*(1), 16–29. https://doi .org/10.1044/2020_JSLHR-19-00190

Magee, M., Lewis, C., Noffs, G., Reece, H., Chan, J. C. S., Zaga, C. J., . . . Vogel, A.P. (2020). Effects of face masks on acoustic analysis and speech perception: Implications for peri-pandemic protocols. *The Journal of the Acoustical Society of America*, *148*(6), 3562–3568. https://doi.org/10.1121/10.0002873

MacLeod, A., & Summerfield, Q. (1990). A procedure for measuring auditory and auditory-visual speech-reception thresholds for sentences in noise: Rationale, evaluation, and recommendations for use. *British Journal of Audiology*, *24*(1), 29–43. https://doi.org/10.3109/03005369009077840

McAuliffe, M. J., Fletcher, A. R., Kerr, S. E., O'Beirne, G. A., & Anderson, T. (2017). Effect of dysarthria type, speaking condition, and listener age on speech intelligibility. *American Journal of Speech-Language Pathology*, *26*(1), 113–123. https://doi.org/10.1044/2016_AJSLP-15-0182

McAuliffe, M. J., Kerr, S. E., Gibson, E. M., Anderson, T., & LaShell, P. J. (2014). Cognitive-perceptual examination of remediation approaches to hypokinetic dysarthria. *Journal of Speech, Language, and Hearing Research*, *57*(4), 1268–1283. https://doi.org/10.1044/2014_JSLHR-S-12-0349

McHenry, M. A. (2011). An exploration of listener variability in intelligibility judgments. *American Journal of Speech-Language Pathology*, *20*(2), 119–123. https://doi.org/10.1044/1058-0360(2010/10-0059)

McHenry, M. A., & Parle, A. M. (2006). Construction of a set of unpredictable sentences for intelligibility testing. *Journal of Medical Speech-Language Pathology*, *14*(4), 269–271.

Metz, D. E., Schiavetti, N., & Sitler, R. W. (1980). Toward an objective description of the dependent and independent variables associated with intelligibility assessments of hearing-impaired adults. In J. D. Subtelny (Ed.), *Speech assessment and speech improvement for the hearing impaired* (pp. 72–81). Alexander Graham Bell Association for the Deaf.

Miller, N. (2013). Measuring up to speech intelligibility. *International Journal of Language & Communication Disorders*, *48*(6), 601–612. https://doi .org/10.1111/1460-6984.12061

Miller, N., Deane, K. H., Jones, D., Noble, E., & Gibb, C. (2011). National survey of speech and language therapy provision for people with Parkinson's disease in the United Kingdom: Therapists' practices. *International Journal of Language & Communication Disorders*, *46*(2), 189–201. https://doi.org /10.3109/13682822.2010.484849

Morris, M., & Haley, K. L. (2011). *Chapel Hill Multilingual Intelligibility Test, Finnish Version (bisyllabic words)*. Center for Aphasia and Related Disorders. https://www.med.unc.edu/ahs/sphs/card/wp-content/uploads /sites/486/2018/02/Finnish.pdf

Muñoz, J., Mendoza, E., Fresneda, M. D., Carballo, G., & Ramirez, I. (2002). Perceptual analysis in different voice samples: Agreement and reliability.

Perceptual and Motor Skills, 94(3), 1187–1195. https://doi.org/10.2466%2Fpms.2002.94.3c.1187

Nilsson, M., Soli, S. D., & Sullivan, J. A. (1994). Development of the Hearing in Noise Test for the measurement of speech reception thresholds in quiet and in noise. *The Journal of the Acoustical Society of America, 95*(2), 1085–1099. https://doi.org/10.1121/1.408469

Patel, R., Usher, N., Kember, H., Russell, S., & Laures-Gore, J. (2014). The influence of speaker and listener variables on intelligibility of dysarthric speech. *Journal of Communication Disorders, 51*, 13–18. https://doi.org/10.1016/j.jcomdis.2014.06.006

Platt, L. J., Andrews, G., Young, M., & Quinn, P. T. (1980). Dysarthria of adult cerebral palsy: I. Intelligibility and articulatory impairment. *Journal of Speech, Language, and Hearing Research, 23*(1), 28–40. https://doi.org/10.1044/jshr.2301.28

Porcaro, C. K., Evitts, P. M., King, N., Hood, C., Campbell, E., White, L., & Veraguas, J. (2020). Effect of dysphonia and cognitive-perceptual listener strategies on speech intelligibility. *Journal of Voice, 34*(5), 806.e7–806.e18. https://doi.org/10.1016/j.jvoice.2019.03.013

Pravasilis, P., & Haley, K. L. (2014). *Chapel Hill Multilingual Intelligibility Test, Greek Version (bisyllabic words)*. Center for Aphasia and Related Disorders. https://www.med.unc.edu/ahs/sphs/card/wp-content/uploads/sites/486/2018/02/Greek.pdf

Salaria, R., & Haley, K. L. (2011). *Chapel Hill Multilingual Intelligibility Test, Hindi Version (disyllabic words)*. Center for Aphasia and Related Disorders. https://www.med.unc.edu/ahs/sphs/card/wp-content/uploads/sites/486/2018/02/Hindi.pdf

Schiavetti, N. (1992). Scaling procedures for the measurement of speech intelligibility. In R. D. Kent (Ed.), *Intelligibility in speech disorders: Theory, measurement and management* (pp. 11–34). John Benjamins. https://doi.org/10.1075/sspcl.1.02sch

Stipancic, K. L., Tjaden, K., & Wilding, G. (2016). Comparison of intelligibility measures for adults with Parkinson's disease, adults with multiple sclerosis, and healthy controls. *Journal of Speech, Language, and Hearing Research, 59*(2), 230–238. https://doi.org/10.1044/2015_jslhr-s-15-0271

Swigert, N. B. (2010). *The source for dysarthria* (2nd ed.). Pro-Ed.

Thiessen, A., & Haley, K. L. (2011). *Chapel Hill Multilingual Intelligibility Test, German Version (monosyllabic words)*. Center for Aphasia and Related Disorders. https://www.med.unc.edu/ahs/sphs/card/wp-content/uploads/sites/486/2018/02/German.pdf

Tikofsky, R. S. (1970). A revised list for the estimation of dysarthric single word intelligibility. *Journal of Speech and Hearing Research, 13*(1), 59–64. https://doi.org/10.1044/jshr.1301.59

Tikofsky, R. S., & Tikofsky, R. P. (1964). Intelligibility measures of dysarthric speech. *Journal of Speech and Hearing Research, 7*(4), 325–333. https://doi.org/10.1044/jshr.0704.325

Tjaden, K., & Liss, J. M. (1995). The influence of familiarity on judgments of treated speech. *American Journal of Speech-Language Pathology, 4*(1), 39–48. https://doi.org/10.1044/1058-0360.0401.39

Tjaden, K., & Wilding, G. E. (2004). Rate and loudness manipulations in dysarthria. *Journal of Speech, Language, and Hearing Research, 47*(4), 766–783. https://doi.org/10.1044/1092-4388(2004/058)

Turner, G. S., Tjaden, K., & Weismer, G. (1995). The influence of speaking rate on vowel space and speech intelligibility for individuals with amyotrophic lateral sclerosis. *Journal of Speech, Language, and Hearing Research, 38*(5), 1001–1013. https://doi.org/10.1044/jshr.3805.1001

Utianski, R. L., Lansford, K. L., Liss, J. M., & Azuma, T. (2011). The effects of topic knowledge on intelligibility and lexical segmentation in hypokinetic and ataxic dysarthria. *Journal of Medical Speech-Language Pathology, 19*(4), 25–36.

Van Riper, C. (1963). *Speech correction: Principles and methods* (4th ed.). Prentice-Hall.

Watterson, T., Lewis, K., Allord, M., Sulprizio, S., & O'Neill, P. (2007). Effect of vowel type of reliability of nasality ratings. *Journal of Communication Disorders, 40*(6), 503–512. https://doi.org/10.1016/j.jcomdis.2007.02.002

World Health Organization. (2001). *International classification of functioning, disability, and health.* https://www.who.int/standards/classifications /international-classification-of-functioning-disability-and-health

Yoho, S. E., & Borrie, S. A. (2018). Combining degradations: The effect of background noise on intelligibility of disordered speech. *The Journal of the Acoustical Society of America, 143*(1), 281–286. https://doi.org/10.1121/1.5021254

Yorkston, K. M., & Beukelman, D. R. (1978). A comparison of techniques for measuring intelligibility of dysarthric speech. *Journal of Communication Disorders, 11*(6), 499–512. https://doi.org/10.1016/0021-9924(78)90024-2

Yorkston, K. M., & Beukelman, D. R. (1981). Communication efficiency of dysarthric speakers as measured by sentence intelligibility and speaking rate. *The Journal of Speech and Hearing Disorders, 46*(3), 296–301. https:// doi.org/10.1044/jshd.4603.296

Yorkston, K. M., & Beukelman, D. R. (1984). *Assessment of Intelligibility of Dysarthric Speech: Manual.* Pro-Ed.

Yorkston, K. M., Beukelman, D. R., Hakel, D., & Dorsey, M. (2007). Sentence Intelligibility Test for Windows [Computer Software]. Madonna Rehabilitation Hospital. https://www.madonna.org/institute/software

Yorkston, K. M., Hammen, V. L., Beukelman, D. R., & Traynor, C. D. (1990). The effect of rate control on the intelligibility and naturalness of dysarthric speech. *The Journal of Speech and Hearing Disorders, 55*(3), 550–560. https://doi.org/10.1044/jshd.5503.550

APPENDIX 4–1

Medical Research Council Institute of Hearing Research Audio-Visual Adaptive Sentence Lists

Lists 2 through 8 and 10 were found to have low predictability (19% to 28%) in a study by Keintz, Bunton, and Hoit (2007).

List 1

1. They moved the furniture.
2. He's wiping the table.
3. He hit his head.
4. The yellow leaves are falling.
5. The cat played with some wool.
6. The bag was very heavy.
7. The towel dripped on the carpet.
8. The bull chased the lady.
9. The man dug his garden.
10. The room has a lovely view.
11. The girl helped in the kitchen.
12. The old shoes were muddy.
13. Father's hiding the presents.
14. The milk boiled over.
15. The neighbor knocked at the door.

List 2

1. He tore his shirt.
2. They finished the jigsaw.
3. She brought her camera.
4. The lady watered her plants.
5. The salt cellar's full.

6. The <u>boy</u> <u>hit</u> his <u>thumb</u>.

7. The <u>mother</u> <u>shook</u> her <u>head</u>.

8. The <u>snow</u> <u>lay</u> on the <u>hills</u>.

9. The <u>father</u> <u>used</u> a <u>towel.</u>

10. The <u>tree</u> was in the <u>back garden.</u>

11. The <u>yacht</u> <u>sailed</u> <u>past</u>.

12. The <u>lady</u> <u>pushed</u> the <u>pram.</u>

13. <u>They're</u> <u>leaving</u> <u>today</u>.

14. The <u>picture</u> <u>hung</u> on the <u>wall</u>.

15. The <u>children</u> <u>sit</u> under the <u>tree</u>.

List 3

1. The <u>lunch</u> was <u>very</u> <u>early</u>.

2. The <u>dirty</u> <u>boy</u> is <u>washing</u>.

3. <u>He</u> <u>hid</u> his <u>money</u>.

4. The <u>curtains</u> were <u>too</u> <u>short</u>.

5. The <u>knife</u> <u>cut</u> the <u>cake</u>.

6. <u>They</u> <u>emptied</u> their <u>pockets</u>.

7. The <u>new</u> <u>shoes</u> were <u>tight</u>.

8. The <u>coat</u> <u>hangs</u> in a <u>cupboard</u>.

9. The <u>sun</u> <u>shone</u> through the <u>clouds</u>.

10. <u>She</u> <u>took</u> her <u>purse</u>.

11. The <u>team</u> <u>lost</u> the <u>match</u>.

12. The <u>shirt</u> <u>caught</u> on a <u>nail</u>.

13. <u>They</u> <u>picked</u> some <u>raspberries</u>.

14. The <u>man</u> <u>climbed</u> the <u>mountain</u>.

15. The <u>lady</u> <u>hurt</u> her <u>arm</u>.

List 4

1. The <u>old</u> <u>clothes</u> were <u>dirty</u>.

2. <u>He</u> <u>carried</u> a <u>stick</u>.

3. <u>She</u> <u>read</u> her <u>book</u>.

4. The <u>new</u> <u>house</u> was <u>empty</u>.

5. The <u>thief</u> <u>brought</u> a <u>ladder</u>.

6. The <u>horse</u> <u>stands</u> by the <u>gate</u>.

7. <u>They're</u> <u>heading</u> for the <u>park</u>.

8. The <u>gardener</u> <u>trimmed</u> the <u>hedge</u>.

9. <u>They're</u> <u>standing</u> <u>up</u>.

10. <u>Someone's</u> <u>hiding</u> in the <u>bushes</u>.

11. The <u>waiter</u> <u>lit</u> the <u>candles</u>.

12. The <u>baker</u> <u>iced</u> the <u>cake</u>.

13. The <u>women</u> <u>slipped</u> on the <u>ice</u>.

14. The <u>small</u> <u>puppy</u> was <u>scared</u>.

15. The <u>lady</u> <u>changed</u> her <u>mind</u>.

List 5

1. The <u>daughter</u> <u>closed</u> the <u>box</u>.

2. <u>He</u> <u>broke</u> into the <u>safe</u>.

3. The <u>doctor</u> <u>carries</u> the <u>bag</u>.

4. The <u>new</u> <u>game</u> was <u>silly</u>.

5. The <u>little</u> <u>boy</u> was <u>tired</u>.

6. <u>They</u> <u>saw</u> the <u>sign</u>.

7. <u>She's</u> <u>wrapping</u> the <u>parcel</u>.

8. The <u>children</u> <u>laughed</u> at the <u>clown</u>.

9. The <u>apple</u> <u>pie</u> was <u>hot</u>.

10. The <u>ship</u> <u>sailed</u> up the <u>river</u>.

11. The <u>house</u> had a <u>lovely</u> <u>garden</u>.

12. The <u>noisy</u> <u>dog</u> is <u>barking</u>.

13. <u>They</u> <u>bought</u> some <u>tickets</u>.

14. The <u>man</u> <u>goes</u> to the <u>bank</u>.

15. The <u>nurse</u> <u>helped</u> the <u>child</u>.

List 6

1. The <u>girl</u> <u>knew</u> the <u>story</u>.
2. <u>He</u> <u>reached</u> for a <u>cup</u>.
3. The <u>lady</u> was <u>quite</u> <u>cross</u>.
4. The <u>rope</u> was <u>too</u> <u>short</u>.
5. <u>She's</u> <u>listening</u> to the <u>radio</u>.
6. The <u>husband</u> <u>cleaned</u> the <u>car</u>.
7. The <u>postman</u> <u>leaned</u> on the <u>fence</u>.
8. The <u>china</u> <u>vase</u> was <u>broken</u>.
9. The <u>other</u> <u>team</u> <u>won</u>.
10. <u>They</u> <u>locked</u> the <u>safe</u>.
11. The <u>leaves</u> <u>dropped</u> from the <u>trees</u>.
12. The <u>men</u> <u>watched</u> the <u>race</u>.
13. The <u>bird's</u> <u>building</u> a <u>nest</u>.
14. The <u>woman</u> <u>called</u> her <u>dog</u>.
15. <u>They're</u> <u>waving</u> at the <u>train</u>.

List 7

1. The <u>cat</u> <u>scratched</u> the <u>chair</u>.
2. <u>She</u> <u>tapped</u> at the <u>window</u>.
3. The <u>man</u> <u>painted</u> the <u>gate</u>.
4. <u>He</u> <u>slid</u> on the floor.
5. <u>They're</u> <u>lifting</u> the <u>box</u>.
6. The <u>woman</u> <u>listened</u> to her <u>friend</u>.
7. The <u>driver</u> <u>hooted</u> his <u>horn</u>.
8. The <u>cake</u> <u>tasted</u> <u>nice</u>.
9. The <u>sailor</u> <u>stood</u> on the <u>deck</u>.
10. The <u>young</u> <u>girls</u> were <u>pretty</u>.
11. <u>They</u> <u>painted</u> the <u>ceiling</u>.
12. The <u>back</u> <u>door</u> was <u>shut</u>.

13. The <u>tree</u> <u>lost</u> its <u>leaves</u>.

14. The <u>boy</u> <u>eats</u> with his <u>fork</u>.

15. The <u>young</u> <u>mother's</u> <u>shopping</u>.

List 8

1. The <u>girl</u> <u>sharpened</u> her <u>pencil</u>.

2. <u>She</u> <u>closed</u> her <u>eyes</u>.

3. The <u>puppy</u> <u>licked</u> his <u>master</u>.

4. The <u>plant</u> <u>grows</u> on the <u>wall</u>.

5. The <u>family's</u> <u>having</u> a <u>picnic</u>.

6. The <u>train</u> <u>arrived</u> on <u>time</u>.

7. <u>They</u> <u>won</u> the <u>game</u>.

8. The <u>lady</u> <u>waited</u> for her <u>husband</u>.

9. The <u>post office</u> was <u>near</u>.

10. <u>They</u> <u>rowed</u> the <u>boat</u>.

11. The <u>old</u> <u>fox</u> was <u>sly</u>.

12. The <u>baby</u> <u>lost</u> his <u>rattle</u>.

13. <u>He</u> <u>dug</u> with his <u>spade</u>.

14. The <u>boiled</u> <u>egg</u> was <u>soft</u>.

15. The <u>two</u> <u>ladies</u> were <u>watching</u>.

List 9

1. The <u>car</u> <u>engine's</u> <u>running</u>.

2. <u>They</u> <u>parked</u> by the <u>station</u>.

3. The <u>lemons</u> were <u>quite</u> <u>bitter</u>.

4. <u>They're</u> <u>cutting</u> the <u>grass</u>.

5. The <u>woman</u> <u>called</u> a <u>doctor</u>.

6. The <u>man</u> <u>shaved</u> with a <u>razor</u>.

7. <u>He</u> <u>tied</u> his <u>shoelaces</u>.

8. The <u>bus</u> is <u>leaving</u> <u>early</u>.

9. <u>She's</u> <u>sewing</u> on a <u>button</u>.

10. The horse kicked the rider.

11. The yellow bananas are ripe.

12. The lady has a fur coat.

13. The cat jumped onto the table.

14. The book sits on the shelf.

15. The boy told a joke.

List 10

1. She sings in the bath.

2. The meat was too tough.

3. The child ate some jam.

4. They're stealing the apples.

5. The children dried the dishes.

6. The paper boy was cheeky.

7. The little car was slow.

8. The bath taps are dripping.

9. They came at Easter.

10. He's wearing a tie.

11. The new towel was clean.

12. The water poured from a jug.

13. The red apples were in a bowl.

14. The bus stopped at the shops.

15. The man drew with a pencil.

APPENDIX 4–2

Hearing in Noise Test Sentence Lists

List 1

1. (<u>A</u>/the) boy fell from (a/<u>the</u>) window.

2. (A/<u>the</u>) wife helped her husband.

3. Big dogs can be dangerous.

4. Her shoes (are/<u>were</u>) very dirty.

5. (A/<u>the</u>) player lost (<u>a</u>/the) shoe.

6. Somebody stole the money.

7. (A/<u>the</u>) fire (<u>is</u>/was) very hot.

8. She's drinking from her own cup.

9. (A/<u>the</u>) picture came from (a/the) book.

10. (A/<u>the</u>) car (is/<u>was</u>) going too fast.

List 2

1. (<u>A</u>/the) boy ran down (a/<u>the</u>) path.

2. Flowers grow in (a/<u>the</u>) garden.

3. Strawberry jam (<u>is</u>/was) sweet.

4. (A/<u>the</u>) shop closes for lunch.

5. The police helped (a/<u>the</u>) driver.

6. She looked in her mirror.

7. (A/<u>the</u>) match fell on (a/<u>the</u>) floor.

8. (A/<u>the</u>) fruit came in (<u>a</u>/the) box.

9. He really scared his sister.

10. (A/<u>the</u>) tub faucet (<u>is</u>/was) leaking.

List 3

1. They heard (<u>a</u>/the) funny noise.

2. He found his brother hiding.

3. (A/<u>the</u>) dog played with (<u>a</u>/the) stick.

4. (A/<u>the</u>) book tells (<u>a</u>/the) story.

5. The matches (<u>are</u>/were) on (a/<u>the</u>) shelf.

6. The milk (<u>is</u>/was) by (a/<u>the</u>) front door.

7. (A/<u>the</u>) broom (<u>is</u>/was) in (a/<u>the</u>) corner.

8. (A/<u>the</u>) new road (<u>is</u>/was) on (a/<u>the</u>) map.

9. She lost her credit card.

10. (A/<u>the</u>) team (<u>is</u>/was) playing well.

List 4

1. (A/<u>the</u>) little boy left home.

2. They're going out tonight.

3. (<u>A</u>/the) cat jumped over (a/<u>the</u>) fence.

4. He wore his yellow shirt.

5. (A/<u>the</u>) lady sits in her chair.

6. He needs his vacation.

7. She's washing her new silk dress.

8. (A/<u>the</u>) cat drank from (a/<u>the</u>) saucer.

9. Mother opened (a/<u>the</u>) drawer.

10. (A/<u>the</u>) lady packed her bag.

List 5

1. (A/<u>the</u>) boy did (<u>a</u>/the) handstand.

2. They took some food outside.

3. The young people (<u>are</u>/were) dancing.

4. They waited for an hour.

5. The shirts (<u>are</u>/were) in (a/<u>the</u>) closet.

6. They watched(<u>a</u>/the) scary moving.

7. The milk (<u>is</u>/was) in (a/<u>the</u>) pitcher.

8. (A/<u>the</u>) truck drove up (a/<u>the</u>) road.

9. (A/<u>the</u>) tall man tied his shoes.

10. (<u>A</u>/the) letter fell on (a/<u>the</u>) floor.

List 6

1. (A/<u>the</u>) silly boy (<u>is</u>/was) hiding.

2. (A/<u>the</u>) dog growled at the neighbors.

3. (<u>A</u>/the) tree fell on (a/<u>the</u>) house.

4. Her husband brought some flowers.

5. The children washed the plates.

· 6. They went on vacation.

7. Mother tied (a/<u>the</u>) string too tight.

8. (A/<u>the</u>) mailman shut (a/<u>the</u>) gate.

9. (<u>A</u>/the) grocer sells butter.

10. (A/<u>the</u>) baby broke his cup.

List 7

1. The cows (<u>are</u>/were) in (a/<u>the</u>) pasture.

2. (A/<u>the</u>) dishcloth (<u>is</u>/was) soaking wet.

3. They (have/<u>had</u>) some chocolate pudding.

4. She spoke to her eldest son.

5. (An/<u>the</u>) oven door (is/<u>was</u>) open.

6. She's paying for her bread.

7. My mother stirred her tea.

8. He broke his leg again.

9. (A/<u>the</u>) lady wore (<u>a</u>/the) coat.

10. The cups (<u>are</u>/were) on (a/<u>the</u>) table.

List 8

1. (A/<u>the</u>) ball bounced very high.

2. Mother cut (a/<u>the</u>) birthday cake.

3. (A/<u>the</u>) football game (<u>is</u>/was) over.

4. She stood near (a/<u>the</u>) window.

5. (A/<u>the</u>) kitchen clock (is/<u>was</u>) wrong.

6. The children helped their teacher.

7. They carried some shopping bags.

8. Someone (<u>is</u>/was) crossing (a/<u>the</u>) road.

9. She uses her spoon to eat.

10. (A/<u>the</u>) cat lay on (a/<u>the</u>) bed.

List 9

1. School got out early today.

2. (A/<u>the</u>) football hit (a/<u>the</u>) goalpost.

3. (A/<u>the</u>) boy ran away from school.

4. Sugar (<u>is</u>/was) very sweet.

5. The two children (<u>are</u>/were) laughing.

6. (<u>A</u>/the) fire truck (<u>is</u>/was) coming.

7. Mother got (<u>a</u>/the) saucepan.

8. (A/<u>the</u>) baby wants his bottle.

9. (A/<u>the</u>) ball broke (a/<u>the</u>) window.

10. There (is/<u>was</u>) a bad train wreck.

List 10

1. (A/<u>the</u>) boy broke (a/<u>the</u>) wooden fence.

2. (An/<u>the</u>) angry man shouted.

3. Yesterday he lost his hat.

4. (A/<u>the</u>) nervous driver got lost.

5. (A/<u>the</u>) cook (<u>is</u>/was) baking (<u>a</u>/the) cake.

6. (A/<u>the</u>) chicken laid some eggs.

7. (A/<u>the</u>) fish swam in (a/<u>the</u>) pond.

8. They met some friends at dinner.

9. (A/<u>the</u>) man called the police.

10. (A/<u>the</u>) truck made it up (a/<u>the</u>) hill.

List 11

1. (A/the) neighbor's boy (has/had) black hair.

2. The rain carne pouring down.

3. (An/the) orange (is/was) very sweet.

4. He took the dogs for a walk.

5. Children like strawberries.

6. Her sister stayed for lunch.

7. (A/the) train (is/was) moving fast.

8. Mother shut (a/the) window.

9. (A/the) bakery (is/was) open.

10. Snow falls in the winter.

List 12

1. (A/the) boy went to bed early.

2. (A/the) woman cleaned her house.

3. (A/the) sharp knife (is/was) dangerous.

4. (A/the) child ripped open (a/the) bag.

5. They had some cold cuts for lunch.

6. She's helping her friend move.

7. They ate (a/the) lemon pie.

8. They (are/were) crossing (a/the) street.

9. The sun melted the snow.

10. (A/the) little girl (is/was) happy.

List 13

1. She found her purse in (a/the) trash.

2. (A/the) table (has/had) three legs.

3. The children waved at (a/the) train.

4. Her coat (is/was) on (a/the) chair.

5. (A/the) girl (is/was) fixing her dress.

6. It's time to go to bed.

7. Mother read the instructions.

8. (A/<u>the</u>) dog (<u>is</u>/was) eating some meat.

9. Father forgot the bread.

10. (A/<u>the</u>) road goes up (<u>a</u>/the) hill.

List 14

1. The fruit (<u>is</u>/was) on the ground.

2. They followed (a/<u>the</u>) garden path.

3. They like orange marmalade.

4. There (are/<u>were</u>) branches everywhere.

5. (A/<u>the</u>) kitchen sink (<u>is</u>/was) empty.

6. The old gloves (<u>are</u>/were) dirty.

7. The scissors (<u>are</u>/were) very sharp.

8. (A/<u>the</u>) man cleaned his suede shoes.

9. (A/<u>the</u>) raincoat (is/<u>was</u>) dripping wet.

10. It's getting cold in here.

List 15

1. (A/<u>the</u>) house (has/<u>had</u>) nine bedrooms.

2. They're shopping for school clothes.

3. They're playing in (a/<u>the</u>) park.

4. Rain (<u>is</u>/was) good for the trees.

5. They sat on (<u>a</u>/the) wooden bench.

6. (A/<u>the</u>) child drank some fresh milk.

7. (A/<u>the</u>) baby slept all night.

8. (A/<u>the</u>) saltshaker (is/<u>was</u>) empty.

9. (A/<u>the</u>) policeman knows the way.

10. The buckets fill up quickly.

List 16

1. He played with his toy train.

2. They're watching (a/<u>the</u>) cuckoo clock.

3. Potatoes grow in the ground.

4. (A/<u>the</u>) girl ran along (a/<u>the</u>) fence.

5. (A/<u>the</u>) dog jumped on (a/<u>the</u>) chair.

6. They finished dinner on time.

7. He got mud on his shoes.

8. They're clearing (a/<u>the</u>) table.

9. Some animals sleep on straw.

10. The police cleared (a/the) road.

List 17

1. Mother picked some flowers.

2. (A/<u>the</u>) puppy played with (a/<u>the</u>) ball.

3. (An/<u>the</u>) engine (<u>is</u>/was) running.

4. (An/<u>the</u>) old woman (<u>is</u>/was) at home.

5. They're watching (a/<u>the</u>) train go by.

6. (An/<u>the</u>) oven (<u>is</u>/was) too hot.

7. They rode their bicycles.

8. (A/<u>the</u>) big fish got away.

9. They laughed at his story.

10. They walked across the grass.

List 18

1. (A/<u>the</u>) boy (is/was) running away.

2. (A/<u>the</u>) towel (<u>is</u>/was) near (a/<u>the</u>) sink.

3. Flowers can grow in (<u>a</u>/the) pot.

4. He's skating with his friend.

5. (A/<u>the</u>) janitor swept (a/<u>the</u>) floor.

6. (A/<u>the</u>) lady washed (a/<u>the</u>) shirt.

7. She took off her fur coat.

8. The match boxes (<u>are</u>/were) empty.

9. (A/<u>the</u>) man (<u>is</u>/was) painting (<u>a</u>/the) sign.

10. (A/<u>the</u>) dog carne home at last.

List 19

1. (A/<u>the</u>) painter uses (<u>a</u>/the) brush.

2. (A/<u>the</u>) family bought (<u>a</u>/the) house.

3. Swimmers can hold their breath.

4. She cut (a/<u>the</u>) steak with her knife.

5. They're pushing an old car.

6. The food (<u>is</u>/was) expensive.

7. The children (<u>are</u>/were) walking home.

8. They (have/<u>had</u>) two empty bottles.

9. Milk comes in (<u>a</u>/the) carton.

10. (A/<u>the</u>) dog sleeps in (<u>a</u>/the) basket.

List 20

1. (A/<u>the</u>) clown (<u>has</u>/had) (<u>a</u>/the) funny face.

2. The bath water (<u>is</u>/was) warm.

3. She injured four of her fingers.

4. He paid his bill in full.

5. They stared at (a/<u>the</u>) picture.

6. (A/<u>the</u>) driver started (a/<u>the</u>) car.

7. (A/<u>the</u>) truck carries fresh fruit.

8. (A/<u>the</u>) bottle (<u>is</u>/was) on (a/<u>the</u>) shelf.

9. The small tomatoes (<u>are</u>/were) green.

10. (A/<u>the</u>) dinner plate (<u>is</u>/was) hot.

List 21

1. They're running past (a/<u>the</u>) house.

2. He's washing his face with soap.

3. (A/<u>the</u>) dog's chasing (a/<u>the</u>) cat.

4. (A/<u>the</u>) milkman drives (<u>a</u>/the) small truck.

5. (A/<u>the</u>) bus leaves before (a/<u>the</u>) train.

6. (A/<u>the</u>) baby (<u>has</u>/had) blue eyes.

7. (A/<u>the</u>) bag fell off (a/<u>the</u>) shelf.

8. They (<u>are</u>/were) coming to dinner.

9. They wanted some potatoes.

10. They knocked on (a/<u>the</u>) window.

List 22

1. (<u>A</u>/the) girl came into (a/<u>the</u>) room.

2. (<u>A</u>/the) field mouse found (a/<u>the</u>) cheese.

3. They're buying some fresh bread.

4. (A/<u>the</u>) machine (*is*/was) noisy.

5. (A/<u>the</u>) rice pudding (<u>is</u>/was) ready.

6. They had a wonderful day.

7. (An/<u>the</u>) exit (is/<u>was</u>) well lit.

8. (A/<u>the</u>) train stops at (a/<u>the</u>) station.

9. He (<u>is</u>/was) sucking his thumb.

10. (A/<u>the</u>) big boy kicked the ball.

List 23

1. The paint dripped on the ground.

2. (A/<u>the</u>) towel fell on (a/<u>the</u>) floor.

3. (A/<u>the</u>) family likes fish.

4. The bananas (are/<u>were</u>) too ripe.

5. He grew lots of vegetables.

6. She argues with her sister.

7. (A/<u>the</u>) kitchen window (is/was) clean.

8. He hung up his raincoat.

9. (A/<u>the</u>) mailman brought (<u>a</u>/the) letter.

10. (A/<u>the</u>) mother heard (a/<u>the</u>) baby.

List 24

1. (A/<u>the</u>) waiter brought (a/<u>the</u>) cream.

2. (A/<u>the</u>) teapot (<u>is</u>/was) very hot.

3. (An/<u>the</u>) apple pie (is/<u>was</u>) good.

4. (A/<u>the</u>) jelly jar (<u>is</u>/was) full.

5. (A/<u>the</u>) girl (is/<u>was</u>) washing her hair.

6. (A/<u>the</u>) girl prayed with (a/<u>the</u>) baby.

7. (A/<u>the</u>) cow (is/<u>was</u>) milked every day.

8. They called an ambulance.

9. They (<u>are</u>/were) drinking coffee.

10. He climbed up (a/<u>the</u>) ladder.

List 25

I. (A/<u>the</u>) boy slipped on the stairs.

2. New neighbors (<u>are</u>/were) moving in.

3. (A/<u>the</u>) girl caught (<u>a</u>/the) head cold.

4. His father will come home soon.

5. (A/<u>the</u>) bus stopped suddenly.

6. He (<u>is</u>/was) washing his car.

7. (A/<u>the</u>) cat caught (<u>a</u>/the) little mouse.

8. They broke all the brown eggs.

9. (A/<u>the</u>) candy shop (<u>is</u>/was) empty.

10. (A/<u>the</u>) lady went to (a/<u>the</u>) store.

Note: Reproduced from Nilsson, M., Soli, S. D., & Sullivan, J. A. (1994). Development of the Hearing in Noise Test for the measurement of speech reception thresholds in quiet and in noise. *The Journal of the Acoustical Society of America*, 95(2), 1085–1099. https://doi.org/10.1121/1.408469, with the permission of the Acoustical Society of America.

APPENDIX 4–3

Checklist for Considerations Related to Assessment of Intelligibility

Checklist for Assessment of Intelligibility	

Speaker Considerations	☐ Choose appropriate assessment for level of severity
	☐ Keep client's rate of speech consistent during assessment
	☐ Record at optimal times for clients considering:
	  ☐ Fatigue level
	  ☐ Effects of medications

Communicative Message Considerations	☐ Select appropriate message for client
	  ☐ Words
	  ☐ Sentences
	  ☐ Paragraph
	  ☐ Narrative
	☐ Choose level of predictability
	  ☐ Predictable message
	  ☐ Unpredictable message

Listener Considerations	☐ Select listener task
	  ☐ Multiple choice
	  ☐ Transcription
	☐ Control for listener experience
	  ☐ Experienced with disordered speech
	  ☐ Inexperienced with disordered speech

Checklist for Assessment of Intelligibility (*continued*)	
	☐ Control for listener familiarity with speaker
	☐ Familiar with speaker
	☐ Unfamiliar with speaker
	☐ Select presentation mode
	☐ Audio-only
	☐ Auditory-Visual
Communication Environment Considerations	☐ Choose recording equipment and use consistently
	☐ Control for mouth to microphone distance
	☐ Select appropriate listening conditions
	☐ Quiet environment
	☐ Naturalistic environment

CHAPTER 5

Speaker Subsystem Management Strategies to Improve Intelligibility

Key Points:

■ Using a framework to guide decision-making can assist in developing a comprehensive management plan for your client.

■ Addressing disorders at the subsystem level can improve overall speech intelligibility.

■ Outcome measures that compare pre versus posttreatment data on clients can take the forms of body/functions, intelligibility, and participation and quality of life.

When you plan management to improve intelligibility, you need to have knowledge of a client's strengths and challenge areas. You have this information if the client has had a thorough evaluation. You want to set functional goals that will allow your client to communicate in the most effective way with the least number of restrictions. Planning treatment activities that involve the client's frequent communication partners and situations is a good way to address functional needs. This chapter begins with a description of frameworks that can guide your management plan for clients. Management strategies related to each of the subsystems with an overall goal of improving intelligibility are addressed.

GUIDING FRAMEWORKS FOR MANAGEMENT DECISIONS

We can use several frameworks to assist with our decision-making about management plans for clients. Clark (2020) provides an excellent overview of several frameworks that can help guide your management decisions for clients. She suggests that knowledge of specific methodologies combined with principles based on these frameworks can help us make the best choices in planning management. Clark describes these frameworks in using treatment for dysarthria, but states they could be useful with other disorders as well.

International Classification of Function

As described in Chapter 1, the ICF (World Health Organization, 2001) allows us to consider the impact of a health problem in more than one way. In planning treatment for a client, we can use the ICF to consider the overall disorder or disease, including complicating factors such as fatigue or cognitive issues that might affect our selection of treatment modalities. It is important to consider the prognosis, specifically whether to expect improvement over time. Sometimes, clients recover function during periods of spontaneous recovery after a stroke. Some clients improve following medical treatment. On the other hand, some clients with reduced intelligibility might have overall health conditions where we anticipate degeneration or worsening conditions. These factors will influence the goals we choose and how frequently we see the client for treatment. Hustad and Weismer (2007) urge clinicians working with patients with dysarthria to consider two intervention pathways. One involves remediation of subsystems, which relates to body functions and structures in ICF; the second addresses reduction of activity limitations and restrictions of participation. A combination of these pathways might be the best choice for most clients.

Using the ICF framework described in Chapter 1, we consider the body functions and structures, including the impairment encountered in muscles, nerves, or subsystems. For example, goals related to respiration or articulation would be related to this portion of the framework and are addressed in this chapter. We would expect limitations in activities and participation restrictions in clients with reduced intelligibility; therefore, having the client's perspective on how their life is affected will help us select functional goals for management. The ICF framework also considers contextual factors, which include personal and environmental factors.

Our selection of goals and materials can be influenced by personal factors, including the client's interests, personality, motivation, and other challenges, like cognitive or language issues. It's a good idea to communicate with the client and family to enlighten yourself about personal factors. Following an accident or diagnosis of a serious illness, many of the personal factors may be different from those in the past (Threats, 2007). People deal differently with these very serious life situations. One client may be extremely motivated, another may feel depressed and not cope well with their disorder. Having good communication with the client and family can help you understand what will improve motivation in treatment. The ICF list of environmental factors includes both facilitators that assist a person's functioning and barriers that limit functioning. Environmental factors can include access to or ability to use technology, as well as support from family, coworkers, and friends. These factors can be modified so they are useful to us in planning management for our clients. Altering environmental factors can include changing the actual communication environment or having the listener learn new strategies to help the client. Management of environmental factors can contribute to improved communication for your client and are discussed in later chapters.

Evidence-Based Practice (EBP)

We use multiple sources in decision-making when we employ EBP. We use the best available evidence from research, along with our own clinical expertise, and the values of our clients and their families. Clark (2020) suggests that use of this model facilitates positive outcomes and client satisfaction. The client is more likely to be happy with outcomes if they have had input into treatment decisions. The client is the "expert" in what they find challenging about their own communication impairment. One serious challenge to the use of EBP is that clinicians find it to be too time consuming, stating that locating the research can be a burden (Mullen, 2005; Zipoli & Kennedy, 2005). As more emphasis has been placed on use of EBP by ASHA and in many graduate programs, investigators have conducted studies to determine if SLPs have found it easier to utilize. Despite the increased education and exposure, recent studies on SLPs use of EBP showed that time and high caseload remain as barriers to the use of EBP (Fulcher-Rood et al., 2020; Greenwell & Walsh, 2021). Solutions are offered by researchers who work together through groups like Division 2 and the Academy of Neurological Communication Disorders and Sciences (ANCDS). Committees were formed to establish guidelines for using EBP in the treatment of dysarthria. Spencer (2006) offers a useful summary to explain this process and direct you to those guidelines. Work settings, such as hospitals and schools are now offering training and journal clubs to help keep up with new findings in the field.

What about clinicians who do not have easy access to a library or online resources to locate journal articles? This is a real problem that may be overlooked by those advocating for the use of EBP. If it's difficult or impossible to locate research, then the use of EBP would be discouraging. ASHA has many resources available to members to help with finding information on current research and thoughts of other clinicians. Table 5–1 contains locations and descriptions of ASHA resources that might be useful in planning treatment using EBP. These resources can provide you with access to updated research, clinical consensus and expertise, as well as studies and guidelines related to clients and their families. There are also resources to guide you through the use of EBP. These resources allow ASHA members to search many topics and find resources created by experts in research and clinical work.

SUBSYSTEM CONTRIBUTION AND MANAGEMENT

This chapter discusses treatment based on the speech subsystems individually and as an interactive unit. During speech, these subsystems do not act independently from each other (Dworkin, 1991). If we use a framework that considers subsystem contributions, we are reminded that speakers need appropriate respiratory support to produce efficient phonation. The articulatory and resonatory systems shape the sounds produced by the combined efforts of the respiratory and phonatory systems. Prosody is affected by all of these subsystems working together. Hustad and Weismer (2007) suggest using a "bottom up" approach to address the respiratory and phonatory systems before working on specific goals for resonance or articulation.

Of course, we want to consider the impairment specifically for each client following evaluation. The topic of subsystem evaluation is covered extensively in Chapter 3; completing this type of evaluation will allow you to know which targets will have greater impact on your particular client's intelligibility. Clinicians often target articulation primarily or exclusively with clients with reduced intelligibility, but this framework suggests that it might be more effective to consider the other subsystems earlier in order to have a greater impact. For example, if respiratory or phonatory issues are noted with a client, addressing articulation before these subsystems might not result in much improvement. Clark (2020) states that her clinical work dictates that prosody may also be an early system to target. In our field, we frequently discuss the subsystems related to dysarthria clients, as many have impairments in more than one subsystem. In considering clients with adult apraxia of speech (AAOS) or voice disorders, there may also be one or more subsystems involved. For any given client, it is a good idea to target the subsystems in a logical order knowing that there is an impact from respiration and phonation on the other subsystems. Many

Table 5–1. Resources for Evidence-Based Practice Available From ASHA

Resource and cost	ASHA Website Location	Description
The EPB Process Free with ASHA membership	https://www.asha.org /research/ebp/evidence -based-practice-process/	Links and information that provide the four steps used in EBP. Deeper dive section with links to guide you through research designs, levels of evidence, and search for evidence.
EBP Toolkit Free with ASHA membership	https://www.asha.org /research/ebp/evidence -based-practice-toolkit/	PDFs that will help you through the process of using EPB. Reference documents: ■ Identify Biases ■ The DECIDE Framework ■ Study Design Features ■ Which Research Design Should you find? Worksheets: ■ Create a PICO Question ■ Create a String Search ■ Track your Search Results
The Practice Portal Free with ASHA membership	https://www.asha.org /practice-portal/	Resources on clinical and professional topics that link to available evidence including: ■ Clinical topics ■ Professional issues ■ Client/Patient handouts ■ Tools and templates More than 40 topics are currently covered, those relevant to reduced intelligibility in adults include: ■ Acquired Apraxia of Speech ■ Dysarthria (Adult) ■ Head and Neck Cancer ■ Voice Disorders

Table 5–1. *continued*

Resource and cost	ASHA Website Location	Description
		All clinical topics cover incidence/prevalence, signs/symptoms, causes, roles/responsibilities, assessment, treatment, resources, and references.
Evidence Maps Free with ASHA membership	https://www2.asha .org/maplanding .aspx?id=8589947062	Online tool created to search terms and find resources, such as guidelines, studies, and reviews which is frequently updated. Maps contain three types of evidence, including: ■ Evidence-based guidelines and systematic reviews of research conducted in topic areas ■ Clinic expertise related to consensus-based statements and ASHA policy documents ■ Client perspectives include individual studies, guidelines and systematic reviews on the perspective of the client and family members
ASHA Special Interest Groups (SIG) Cost is $45 per year for each SIG for ASHA members, $10 for students who are members of NSSLHA or ASHA	https://www.asha.org /sig/	Membership in a SIG allows access to: ■ Online scholarly review journal, Perspectives of the ASHA Special Interest Groups ■ Online SIG Community where members post questions, collaborations, and share resources and knowledge There are 19 SIGs. Those most relevant to topics covered in this book include: ■ SIG 2, Neurogenic Communication Disorders ■ SIG 3, Voice and Upper Airway Disorders ■ SIG 15, Gerontology

Source: American Speech-Language-Hearing Association (n.d.).

behavioral management tasks will be described in this chapter, but readers will find more detailed information in Duffy's 2019 textbook. Additionally, Swigert's 2010 book contains helpful descriptions and explanations of many treatment strategies based on the subsystems.

Respiration

It is critical to note that the respiratory system works together with the phonatory system to produce voice. If the client's respiratory system isn't functioning in the most effective way, the phonatory output or voicing may not be well supported. Not all SLPs feel knowledgeable about the respiratory system; perhaps we have more clinical experience working with other subsystems such as articulation. However, if our client's inefficient respiration can be improved, some clients may have much better speech production. We have some excellent resources in our field and can also rely on our colleagues in respiratory therapy who can provide respiratory measures and assistance. Duffy (2019) reminds us that to improve speech breathing, respiratory exercises should be done during speech production for the most functional results. However, if you are working with a client who is not able to generate enough subglottal pressure to produce voice, work on respiration without phonation may be needed (Spencer et al., 2003).

Diaphragmatic-Abdominal Breathing

According to Boone and colleagues (2019), most people use thoracic breathing, which involves expanding the thorax and contracting the diaphragm during inhalation and doing the opposite during exhalation. These authors, along with many others, advocate for the use of diaphragmatic breathing, which is commonly used by trained voice users and singers. Swigert (2010) suggests having the client lay down on their back in the supine position with one hand on the chest and one on the abdomen. We then ask the client to breathe and feel the rising movement of the hand on the abdomen. Stemple and colleagues (2014) suggest placing a book on the client's abdomen so when they take a breath, they will see the book rise. Encourage clients to practice this type of breathing in supine and upright positions and also during speech production. Starting with simple tasks, like sustained vowels may be a useful way to move from breathing exercises to speech breathing.

Increasing Upper Body Tone

If muscle tone in the upper body and diaphragm are increased, clients may have better control of exhalation and improved respiratory drive for speech (Duffy, 2019). Ask the client to sit in a chair and either push down or pull up on the seat to increase upper body muscle tension. This task can be completed in a wheelchair or the client can push one fist into the other hand. Swigert (2010) suggests using this along with diaphragmatic-abdominal breathing, initially while exhaling and later during phonation.

Body Positioning

In most circumstances, an upright position is best for effective use of air for while speaking. A client, who is slumped over, possibly due to weakness or their position in a wheelchair, may have better respiratory support if we can get them into a more upright position. If they can change positions themselves, verbal instructions and reminders may be helpful. Some clients may need cushions or pads to help them stay more upright and occupational or physical therapists may be helpful in this effort. Research in our field has led to some specific considerations regarding certain diseases and body positions. Clients who have more weakness in exhalation than inhalation may have better respiratory control for speech in the supine position because gravity will provide extra force to push against the diaphragm and move air out. Researchers have noted this in individuals with traumatic brain injury (TBI), multiple sclerosis (MS), and spinal cord injury (Yorkston et al., 2010). Individuals with ALS may have better respiratory control in the upright position, as gravity helps lower the diaphragm into the abdomen while they inhale (Putnam & Hixon, 1984). For any client, you can research the best positioning to determine what is the most effective and functional position.

Controlling Exhalation

We can teach clients to control the length of an exhalation during phonation, which may increase respiratory capacity and improve control of exhaled airstream used for speech (Duffy, 2019). Clients can count, read, or speak naturally while practicing longer and longer exhalations. If they are speaking, you can use a stopwatch to record how long they speak on one exhalation. You should watch for their loudness or voice decreasing if they lose respiratory power near the end of sentences. A sound pressure level (SPL) meter or app that measures intensity could also be used. Some clients may begin to use a glottal fry if they are pushing for a longer utterance and running out of air, so you will want to ensure that the longer controlled exhalations during speech do not result in poor voicing habits.

Another way to assist clients in controlling exhalation is to help them practice speaking immediately at the onset of exhalation. Some clients may take a deep breath, possibly with reminders from you, and then exhale part of it before they begin to speak. In this case, they may still not have adequate respiratory support for speech. Swigert (2010) suggests asking the client to begin phonating a speech sound as soon as exhalation begins with their hand on their abdomen to feel the movement exhalation. Practicing this coordination of breathing with onset of phonation can help the client learn to use air more effectively for speech.

Generating Appropriate Loudness Levels

Inadequate respiratory support may cause reduced loudness. If loudness is affecting your client's intelligibility, you may want to target increasing loudness. Boone et al. (2019) suggest discussing the soft voice with the client and ask them to use a louder voice to determine if they can. An SPL meter or app can help the client visualize their loudness level (see Chapter 3). Although not a respiratory strategy, amplification can be helpful in increasing loudness, but remember that every part of the speech signal will be amplified. If your client has a quiet voice but also has resonance and articulation difficulties contributing to intelligibility, unless we address the other issues, listeners will just hear a louder version of the unintelligible speech.

Muscle Strength Training

Muscle strength training related to respiratory muscles has been investigated in terms of speech and swallowing. Sapienza and Hoffman (2022) describe the two key principles that guide strength training. They mention that the exercise stimulus must be intense enough to change muscle function, which involves the amount of load and the duration of the exercise. The frequency of the exercise is another important principle.

There are two types of strength training related to respiration, one related to inhalation/inspiration, and one related to exhalation/expiration. Inspiratory muscle strength training (IMST) is used to increase inspiratory muscle force. We speak on exhalation, but having an effective inhalation is needed as well. We might use IMST when we want our client to strength train using a strong, quick inhalation and a slow, controlled exhalation (Sapienza & Troche, 2012). Expiratory muscle strength training (EMST) is used to increase expiratory muscle force and involves setting the resistance of the device at 75% of the maximum expiratory pressure the client can achieve (Sapienza & Troche, 2012). Laciuga and colleagues (2014) created a systematic review of research related to EMST, which showed that the participants in several small studies exhibited improved functions in breathing following EMST treatment. Researchers who are studying muscle strength training feel that improved voice quality and speech intelligibility will be outcomes of its use, but we need further investigations to confirm this.

Using Optimal Breath Groups

Some clients do not take breaths at appropriate places when they are speaking. We can teach clients to use optimal breath groups, which basically means taking breaths before the air runs out and you can't produce words. An optimal breath group is the number of syllables that a person can comfortably produce on one breath (Duffy, 2019). Please notice that the word optimal does not refer to more breaths. Work with your client to determine how many syllables they can produce, then practice using that number, so they have enough breath support to complete their words and sentences. Your client can also learn to feel when they are nearly out of air and take breaths when needed, but also consider natural syntactic breaks for pauses, such as between phrases or sentences. Hopefully, using some of the other strategies mentioned in this chapter will allow them to have more syllables per breath. However, if that isn't possible or takes time, this is a good strategy to allow listeners to hear all syllables and words that the client produces.

Inspiratory Checking

When a person takes a deep breath, their lungs will recoil or snap back into place with greater force than a smaller breath. In a client who has a weak respiratory system, this can cause listeners to hear bursts of loudness and wasted air (Duffy, 2019). For these clients, it is helpful to teach them to maintain a steady pressure while speaking (Netsell, 1998). Have the client inhale to about 50% of their maximum lung capacity and then slowly let the air out while speaking. Using this technique can lead to more syllables per breath group and increased intelligibility in clients with dysarthria (Netsell, 1998).

Phonation

The phonatory system works normally if the respiratory system is functioning effectively. The previous section stated the importance of completing respiratory tasks during phonation. During phonatory tasks, we will also want to ensure the client is using effective respiration. We may see reduced intelligibility as a result of phonation issues related to dysarthria or voice disorders. Even if a client has only a phonatory disorder, intelligibility can be reduced (Evitts et al., 2016; Porcaro et al., 2019). Information from a thorough voice evaluation will allow you to determine what targets to select for phonation goals. Thomas and Stemple (2007) created a review of research related to treatment of voice disorders. These authors wrote about three different approaches to voice disorders, including symptom-based, physiologically based, and vocally hygienic treatment. This article is recommended, along with *The Source for Dysarthria* (Swigert, 2010) and voice disorder textbooks, such as those by Boone et al. (2019), and Sapienza and Hoffman (2022). These sources provide details and more options, but samples of voice management techniques that might be useful with clients who have reduced intelligibility are included here.

Using Effortful Closure

Clients who have breathy voices with reduced loudness may benefit from using techniques that increase the closure of the vocal folds. Keep in mind, there can be various reasons for breathiness. For example, a client who has vocal nodules may have a breathy, soft voice, but with this client, we would not want to use effortful closure techniques as overuse or hyperadduction of the vocal folds likely caused the nodules. This is yet another reminder that gaining information about the cause or physiology is just as important as knowing how the client sounds perceptually. Getting an evaluation from an ENT is a critical step with voice clients. The suggested techniques here would apply to clients who are not achieving good vocal fold closure due to weakness or paralysis, which may include clients diagnosed with voice disorders or dysarthria. Stemple and colleagues (2014) describe methods that can be used safely and effectively to improve vocal fold closure. You can teach the client to use a hard glottal attack by producing a sharp phonation. Use of hard glottal attack as a primary approach to therapy has the potential to lead to vocal hyperfunction, so its use can help a client achieve the sensation of having adequate vocal fold closure (Stemple et al., 2014). These authors also recommend the use of pushing down or pulling up on the seat to increase upper body tension and improve vocal fold closure. When teaching the client to increase glottal closure, be sure you are not teaching them constant use of strain or hyperfunctional voice behaviors, such as tension in neck muscles or they may experience other types of voice problems. Finding the middle ground is key.

Timing Phonation With Exhalation

Clients with vocal fold weakness and possible incoordination between the respiratory and phonatory systems could benefit from practice on timing of phonation (Duffy, 2019). Starting phonation immediately after inhalation can help minimize air wastage and may contribute to a louder voice with longer phonation time. Start by using sustained vowels, words, and then build up to longer utterances.

Low Impact Voicing

Using confidential voice can be helpful when you want clients to adopt a softer, easy onset voice (Colton & Casper, 1996). Confidential voice involves using a light, breathy voice, as if you are in a room where you do not want other people nearby to hear what you say. This can be helpful for clients who have too much tension and have a harsh or tense sounding voice. Low impact voicing reduces loudness and abusive vocal patterns (Behrman et al., 2008). Teachers who used amplification along with confidential voice reported more clarity in their speech and more ease in voice production (Roy et al., 2001). You do not want your client to whisper, as a whisper is not actual phonation and can cause strain on the vocal folds (Boone, 2019).

Utilizing Relaxation Techniques

Sapienza and Hoffman (2022) describe mindfulness-based stress reduction (MBSR) strategies that assist clients in using breathwork and meditation to improve awareness of tension in the body. These techniques can be useful for clients with increased tension, including muscle tension dysphonia. Voice symptoms related to stress in the body include diplophonia, elevated pitch, harshness, and shortness of breath (Boone, 1997). There are many instructional materials and videos on the topic of relaxing the body. You can teach your client to use total body relaxation or focus more on the laryngeal area. These strategies often involve being in a quiet place, focusing on breathing and tensing, then relaxing muscles. In some clients, excess laryngeal tension may occur because of poor respiratory support or poor coordination between respiration and phonation. In these cases, some of the respiratory management techniques previously mentioned may be useful. If you are working with a client whose voice is impacted by excess tension, teaching them to speak in a more relaxed manner with strong respiratory support will be a functional, beneficial target.

Speaking With High Phonatory Effort

Clients who have reduced intelligibility related to breathy voice and low loudness level can benefit from several programs where the goal is to use a higher phonatory effort level when speaking. By increasing phonatory effort, these programs serve as voice strengthening programs which can improve other aspects, including prosody and intelligibility.

Lee Silverman Voice Treatment (LSVT®) is a well-researched voice program which requires SLPs to participate in training that leads to certification. The focus of LSVT is on learning how to use loud voice and high speech effort, while the clinician teaches the client to calibrate their own loudness level and self-regulate as needed. There are many investigations showing the effectiveness of LSVT for people with Parkinson's disease (Cannito et al., 2012; Ramig et al., 1995). Mahler and colleagues (2015) found improved function in speech rate, monotone, voice quality, and speech intelligibility, with effects lasting up to two years. The LSVT website, found at https://www.lsvtglobal.com/ contains information on the training/certification process and lists of the many investigations of LSVT in different populations of children and adults.

The Parkinson Voice Project has created voice therapy programs for individuals with Parkinson's disease called SPEAK OUT!® and LOUD Crowd®. Prior to using these programs with clients, SLPs must complete training.

SPEAK OUT! is the first step in the training where the client takes part in individual sessions where the focus is to learn how to speak with intent. Following completion of that program (typically 12 sessions), the client attends LOUD Crowd sessions, which is a group maintenance program that continues use of the same speech targets. Research on these programs has found that individuals with Parkinson's disease show improved vocal loudness, reading intelligibility, and voice quality (Behrman et al., 2020; Boutsen et al., 2018). For further information on SPEAK OUT! and LOUD Crowd training and research, you can visit the Parkinson Voice Project website at https://www.parkinsonvoiceproject.org/

Phonation Resistance Training Exercises (PhoRTE)

Ziegler and Hapner (2013) developed PhoRTE to assist individuals who are experiencing age-related voice changes. This program has a less intensive schedule than LSVT or SPEAK OUT! and focuses on individuals with presbyphonia (aging voice) rather than Parkinson's disease. PhoRTE sessions focus on both loudness and pitch variation during phonation using resistance strength training principles. The four-step process involved in using PhoRTE with clients is available in Zeigler and Hapner's descriptive article. Adults with presbyphonia were found to have shown reduced vocal effort in combination with increased satisfaction with their voice-related quality of life (Zeigler et al., 2014). PhoRTE combined with EMST was found to improve voice outcomes in individuals with presbyphonia (Belsky et al., 2021).

Using Holistic Voice Therapy Programs

Several programs have been developed to manage voice disorders by involving multiple subsystems. Two programs are commonly mentioned in voice disorders textbooks that utilize respiratory, phonatory, and resonatory systems in the same tasks. These programs have been developed to instruct clients to use safe vocal behaviors while improving voice quality. Stemple and colleagues (2014) recommend both for a wide variety of voice disorders, including hyperfunctional and hypofunctional disorders.

Vocal function exercises (VFE) were first described by Barnes (1977) and modified by Stemple et al. (2014). VFE is a systematic exercise program that involves respiratory, laryngeal, and resonance activities to achieve the best voice with the least amount of effort. The program starts by describing the voice problem to the client using visuals and then teaching them to complete a series of exercises to practice twice a day at home. VFE was shown to be effective in speakers with normal voices (Stemple et al., 1994) teachers with voice disorders (Roy et al., 2001), trained singers (Sabol et al., 1995) and elderly men (Gorman, 2000). The program can be useful for clients who desire or need a regimented program to follow. A complete description of the program's steps can be found in a clinical voice textbook by Stemple and colleagues (2014) and a book and practice DVD (Stemple, 2011) are also available from Plural Publishing, at https://www.pluralpub lishing.com/publications/vocal-function-exercises.

Lessac-Madsen Resonant Voice Therapy (LMRVT) was developed by Verdolini Abbott (2008a, 2008b, 2008c) based on concepts from two voice experts, Arthur Lessac and Mark Madsen. The idea behind LMRVT is for the client to use easy, gentle phonation along with increased awareness of oral vibratory sensations. What the patient feels and hears of their own voice is a critical component. LMRVT is a fairly new program and studies of resonant voice therapy techniques have shown some improvements, but controlled, long-term studies are needed to support its use. Yiu and colleagues (2017) completed a helpful systematic review which lists the outcomes of studies related to resonant voice therapy. LMRVT exercises are described in good detail in several voice textbooks, including those by Stemple and colleagues (2014) and Sapienza and Hoffman (2022). Verdolini Abbott (2008a, 2008b, 2008c) has created a manual for the SLP, a manual for the patient, and a DVD to help clinicians utilize this program. You can find these at https://www.pluralpublishing.com/publications /lessac-madsen-resonant-voice-therapy-clinician-manual.

Implementing Vocal Hygiene

If you are working with a voice client who has some unhealthy vocal behaviors that caused a voice disorder or has developed some because of the disorder, teaching them about vocally hygienic behaviors is necessary since this can contribute to reduced intelligibility (Evitts et al, 2016; Porcaro et al., 2019). Pannbacker and Hayes (2008) completed a systematic review of voice treatment in teachers, a profession where there are frequent voice disorders. They reported that in recent studies where teachers received voice treatment, vocal hygiene was the most frequently used treatment method and was included in five of the 10 studies reviewed. Vocal hygiene was found to improve vocal function and use in teachers in combination with other treatment methods (Bovo et al., 2007; Roy et al., 2001) as well as in isolation (Chan, 1994; Duffy & Hazlett, 2004). In reading literature related to voice treatment, it is important to know what is being examined, prevention versus treatment and how measures are made, instrumental versus perceptual or client report of symptoms. The review by Pannbaker and Hayes (2008) is a helpful resource, as they provide analysis on the types and strengths of studies related to vocal hygiene among teachers. Sapienza and Hoffman (2022) suggest that vocal hygiene should be used in combination with other treatment strategies that address improved laryngeal function specific to your client's disorder.

Individuals with professions or activities that require heavy voice use are not the only people who can benefit from vocally hygienic practices.

SLPs should counsel clients with dysarthria and AAOS on safe voice use and strategies. Stemple and colleagues (2014) provide a 4-step vocal hygiene plan, which includes:

1. Identify the traumatic behavior. Interview the client to determine if they have any current behaviors that might cause trauma to the vocal fold tissue, including shouting, throat clearing, coughing, laryngeal muscle strain, and lack of appropriate hydration.

2. Describe the effect. Use videos and illustrations to educate the client about how the vocal folds work, and the impact of lesions or strain on the voice. If the client has seen an ENT and had a stroboscopic evaluation, you can show them their own vocal folds. Understanding how a behavior can damage the vocal fold tissue is often a motivating factor in helping clients change behaviors.

3. Define specific occurrences. Ask the client to describe how they use their voice on a typical day. They may not realize how much they are talking or what activities might put their voice at risk. Activities like church choir, teaching an aerobics class, or a long phone call with a friend may not seem problematic, but it is a good idea to discuss all voice use to see what can be modified.

4. Change traumatic vocal behavior. This step will involve discussion about any behaviors you find that might contribute to poor vocal hygiene. Some are more general, such as increasing hydration. Most people think that all fluids they are consuming are providing hydration, but this is not the case. Alcohol and caffeinated beverages are drying to the tissues in the larynx. If someone is drinking large amounts of caffeinated beverages, they are not increasing hydration and they may feel too full to consume the water that they need. Stemple and colleagues (2014) remind us that the appropriate amount of hydration will vary by the person's body size and physical activity, but their textbook includes two common recommendations. The first is drinking eight 8 oz. glasses of water per day and the second is drinking half the person's body weight in ounces. If you do not feel comfortable telling the client a specific amount, you can stress the importance of them having a conversation with their physician on this topic.

   Some modifications will be more closely related to vocal use and the behaviors you have identified with the client as potentially abusive. Overuse of the voice can be addressed by discussion with the client on when they can take voice naps or rest. Targeting times when they do not have to use their voice in their regular schedule can be helpful. Perhaps they can use their drive into work as a voice rest time rather than calling someone or singing along with the radio. Modification of vocal behaviors is specific to each client and what they will change. It is helpful to provide alternative behaviors rather than just asking them to stop behaviors that are part of their daily functioning. For example, a teacher or coach could use a whistle or hand clap to gain attention rather than yelling. There may be times when they could send an e-mail or text rather than calling someone for a lengthy phone call. If post-nasal drip is contributing to coughing or throat-clearing, seeing an ENT may eliminate the cause of these behaviors. It's a good idea to work closely with your client so help them understand the impact of any potential vocally abusive behaviors and then help reinforce changes that are needed.

Enhancing Loudness With Prosthetics

For clients whose reduced loudness leads to lower intelligibility, there are some prosthetic options that may be helpful. Several devices have been developed to help monitor voice parameters, including fundamental frequency and intensity. These devices can provide feedback to clients who may have targets related to pitch and loudness. Carryover of new voice behaviors to the client's daily life can be one of the more difficult aspects of voice management (Ziegler, 2014) and these devices may be of use, although investigations are needed. Nacci and colleagues (2013) discussed the use of the Ambulatory Phonation Monitor, developed by KayPENTAX, with a group of teachers with dysphonia, although investigations in its use have not been completed. Another device, the Voice Health Monitor, has been used in an investigation of client feedback in cases with vocal nodules as an early step toward providing evidence of its functional use (Van Stan et al., 2017). Use of the VoxLog®, another feedback device, has been investigated to establish optimal parameters for use with people with Parkinson's disease (Gustafsson, 2016).

When normal speakers are in a noisy environment, their loudness typically increases, which is called the Lombard effect. The SpeechVive is a device that was developed to take advantage of this and has been effective in speakers with Parkinson's disease. It is a small wearable device that plays multi-talker babble noise in one ear. Huber and colleagues (2019) reported improved vocal intensity and length of utterance in speakers with Parkinson's disease after eight weeks of SpeechVive use. These types of devices may prove useful for individuals who require feedback and cues to maintain voice parameters, such as increased intensity to improve intelligibility.

Resonance

As discussed in Chapter 2, resonance issues can impact intelligibility by increasing or decreasing nasality. Hyponasality occurs when there is limited nasal coloring of the nasalized sounds (m, n, and ŋ) and usually involves a medical referral to determine the cause and potential treatment. Hypernasality occurs when there is too much nasality and can vary in severity. There are multiple reasons for hypernasality, so determining the cause is important. Causes of hypernasality in adults include slow or weak movements of the velum and reduced control over coordination between the velum and posterior/lateral walls of the pharynx. Lack of closure of the velopharyngeal port can also impact articulation. Velopharyngeal incompetency can reduce a speaker's ability to build up pressure for sounds such as plosives, fricatives, and affricates (i.e., the pressure consonants). Assisting clients with resonance can be challenging as they cannot see their velum or move it voluntarily in isolation. It is not as simple as instructing a client about lip or tongue placement. Medical approaches, including surgery (e.g., a pharyngeal flap), or use of prosthetics, such as a palatal lift or obturator, can be useful. If you feel a client's nasality is affecting their intelligibility, a referral to an ENT may be a first step in the process of determining if a medical approach will benefit your client. It may be helpful to have the client read the same passage normally and again with the nostrils pinched with fingers or a nose clip. This will allow you to hear how any changes in intelligibility are noted before deciding on a medical referral. Regardless of the type of management you plan, please read Yorkston and colleagues (2001) for a summary of evidence-based practices related to dysarthria compiled by experts in this area. Duffy (2019) reminds us that what we know about behavioral management of velopharyngeal inadequacy comes largely from expert opinion as opposed to evidence from research studies. Guidelines based on evidence in this area point to behavioral strategies that focus on four major areas (Yorkston et al., 2001).

1. Modifying speech patterns
    Duffy (2019) explains that these techniques do not concentrate directly on velopharyngeal movements, or function, but may influence it through the speaker's efforts in related areas. Swigert (2010) mentions that these activities will not improve velopharyngeal function but may reduce the perception of hypernasality. Speech pattern modifications might include overarticulation, which involves exaggeration of jaw and mouth movements. Swigert (2010) recommends helping the client to hear the difference between hypernasal and normal resonance by having them listen to examples of nasal and non-nasal sentences. Then, adding the over-articulation using a mirror to observe the larger mouth and jaw movements. Reducing the speaker's rate may improve intelligibility (see Chapter 6) and may reduce listener's perception of hypernasality (Duffy, 2019; Swigert, 2010).
    Techniques that aim to change vocal behaviors to optimize the flow of air can also be helpful in improving resonance. Clients

who have thin, front focus voice, a voice focused in the back of the mouth, or lower in the throat can change the focus of the voice. Stemple and colleagues (2019) define "focus" as where the voice is resonating in the airways. Correct focus of the voice comes from the middle of the mouth, as opposed to being trapped in the pharyngeal area. Use of forward or frontal focus can be a helpful technique for clients who use a tongue position that is too far forward or backward in the mouth, making the oral-pharyngeal resonance unbalanced. Sapienza and Hoffman (2022) suggest giving the client the direction to "move the voice from the back of the throat to the front of the mouth while feeling vibrations in the nasal cavity" (p. 243). Instruct the client to think about a mask surrounding their eyes and nose, and that the area of the mask is the ideal area for the voice to resonate. Boone et al. (2019) provide a multistep process for using frontal focus strategies with clients. Several studies have shown that voice improvement happens quickly when the client changes the focus of their voice, using techniques related to resonance, such as VFE (Bane et al., 2019; Dargin et al., 2016).

2. Training for resistance
   Individuals who have sleep apnea often sleep with a continuous positive airway pressure (CPAP) device that delivers positive pressure into the nasal cavities through a mask. Positive impacts on hypernasality and intelligibility have been noted when CPAP is used during speech training tasks with clients following traumatic brain injury (Cahill et al., 2004; Kuehn & Wachtel, 1994). The muscle which elevates the velum (levator veli palatini) was shown to work harder with increasing levels of nasal air pressure in clients with and without cleft palates (Kuehn et al., 1993). We need more evidence with larger studies of different disorders, but use of CPAP during speech practice is showing potential. For a review of the theory behind its use, see Liss et al. (1994).

3. Some speakers may improve nasality if feedback is used to help them see or feel where the airflow is directed (Duffy, 2019). Feedback on nasality could come in high-tech form, such as a nasometer, which allows the client to see the amount of oral versus nasal resonance during speech. See Watterson (2020) for a helpful review of nasometer use, and how to interpret nasalance scores. For less expensive, low tech options, some clinicians use the See-Scape™ (Pro-Ed), which can be used to indicate movement of nasal airflow or a mirror placed under the client's nostril where moisture or fogging will indicate airflow movement from the nose.

4. You may see nonspeech activities, tools, and tasks that are promoted to improve resonance. These techniques, including pushing, blowing

cotton balls, or whistles, sucking, icing and stroking, have not been effective in improving resonance during speech (Yorkston et al., 2001).

Articulation

Traditional methods of articulation therapy were initially discussed by Rosenbek and LaPointe (1985). These methods are commonly suggested as approaches to improve articulation and, therefore, intelligibility in adults (Duffy, 2019; Freed, 2020; Swigert, 2010). The three identified traditional methods include integral stimulation, phonetic placement, and phonetic derivation. Integral stimulation involves tasks where the client watches and listens to the clinician and then imitates the model. Phonetic placement involves the use of models, illustrations, and hands-on assistance for the client to achieve the correct targets and movements of the articulators. In some cases, the client may require the SLP to physically move articulators into place. Phonetic derivation occurs when we use a sound or movement the client can accomplish to help them produce a sound they do not produce correctly.

Other techniques can be utilized to improve articulatory skills. Minimal contrasts can be very useful in working on consonants (Duffy, 2019). These contrasts include word pairs such as "may-bay," "school-cool," or "kick-thick." When you use minimal pairs, it is important that you explain to the client that the idea behind this approach is to make them sound distinctly different. Although it can be tricky to come up with your own words, there are many resources for minimal pair word lists, including the one on the CD of treatment materials provided by Swigert (2010).

If we want to improve intelligibility, it is critical that we choose targets based on their contribution to the client's intelligibility (Duffy, 2019). We should also consider if the client can produce the sounds at syllable, word, or sentence levels when we set target goals. It is preferred to use real words, rather than nonsense words. Intelligibility drills can improve skills in articulation, rate, and prosody (Yorkston et al., 2010). An intelligibility drill involves the client reading words or sentences or describing pictures to a listener who does not know what they are saying. These types of drills can be useful because the client receives feedback from the listener about what was misunderstood and what was heard instead. They can then use that information to revise their production. Duffy (2019) reminds us that this type of task can be adjusted to different levels of difficulty to help the client achieve some level of intelligibility. Many clients with dysarthria have learned compensatory movements and allowing them to be used and modified, if needed, can improve intelligibility. In some of these cases, the client may produce an approximation of a word or sound and if it's acceptable and leads to the listener understanding, this can be reinforced. If the listener doesn't understand the approximation, the client will need to adjust further.

Clark (2020) points out articulation treatments may be overused with clients with dysarthria. She reveals two reasons why this might be the case. First, errors of articulation are common in all dysarthria types and are fairly easy to detect during an evaluation. For these reasons, articulation may be an obvious target. She also states that SLPs commonly receive thorough training and, therefore, may feel more comfortable with articulation treatment than those directed at other subsystems. In considering the bottom-up approach mentioned earlier, goals targeting respiration, phonation, and resonation should be considered when applicable for clients prior to articulation goals. Clark notes that she has seen improved articulation skills when these other subsystems are addressed along with articulation. She cautions against treating articulation in isolation and reminds us to consider the interaction between the subsystems.

Modifying Habitual Speech: Clear and Loud Speech

The idea of clear speech involves providing instructions, cues, and possibly models for speakers to modify their habitual speech. When given directions to modify how they habitually speak, people can change their typical manner of speech. Instructions for what defines clear speech varies among these studies, but involves use of cues such as, "slow down," "overenunciate," or "exaggerate movements of your mouth." Loud speech may involve cues such as, "speak as if your listener is hearing impaired" or "speak like you are talking in a very noisy background." The idea behind clear speech is not to give specific instructions but rather to have the client modify in their own way, after receiving general directions.

Many studies have shown that clear speech instructions can modify how people speak, but most have used non-disordered speakers. Several studies have included speakers with dysarthria and those findings indicate that intelligibility is improved by using clear speech. Beukelman and colleagues (2002) investigated use of clear speech in individuals following TBI and found that clear speech cues and models improved intelligibility by 8%. It is interesting that this 8% increase in intelligibility did not reach statistical significance but that 8% would surely make a functional difference in a client's life. Research aimed at speakers with Parkinson's disease and multiple sclerosis showed that both clear and loud instruction resulted in higher intelligibility compared to habitual speech (Tjaden et al., 2013; Tjaden et al., 2014). Because these studies demonstrated improved intelligibility in individuals with dysarthria, you may want to adapt the methods used in these studies with your clients. For the loud speech condition, individuals were instructed to speak twice as loud as their regular speaking voice and were cued about speaking as though they were talking to someone in a noisy environment or who had a hearing loss. For the clear condition, they were instructed to speak twice as clearly as their typical speech, with cues to exaggerate mouth movements. We've also learned that directions to speak clearly related to over enunciation or exaggerated mouth movements lead clients to focus on modifying their articulation, while directions related to speaking as those talking to someone with a hearing impairment result in changes to pitch and loudness (Lam & Tjaden, 2016). These different approaches may be helpful when working with clients as you can target their modification to the subsystem(s) that you feel will have the most impact on intelligibility. For an interesting study on an intensive treatment program based on clear speech with dysarthria related to TBI and stroke, see Park et al. (2016).

Deciding on Use of Nonspeech Oral Motor Exercises (NSOME)

The use of nonspeech exercises to strengthen musculature to move articulatory structures (lips, tongue, jaw), laryngeal and respiratory muscles is common in the field of speech-language pathology (Lof & Watson, 2008). Clinicians often write goals to increase strength when using NSOME. Studies have shown that we do not need full strength of the articulators to produce speech. Lip muscle force during speech is only about 10% to 20% of the maximal capabilities for lip force, and only about 11% to 15% of the available jaw force is used during speech (Bunton & Weismer, 1994). A heavy focus on strength without consideration to other movement factors, including timing, accuracy of articulator movement to the target position, and similar factors, would not be expected to improve speech production. In addition, there are some clients where strengthening exercises may create more problems. Any type of strengthening exercises are contraindicated for clients with myasthenia gravis or some clients with disease with expected rapid degeneration, rigidity, or spasticity of speech musculature (Duffy, 2019).

Many reviews of terminology, use, and motor principles have been written to help clinicians understand how to work with clients who have movement-related speech disorders. Please read the summaries and reviews written by clinical and research experts in motor speech disorders on this topic, including Clark (2003), Kent (2015), and McCauley et al. (2009). A systematic review of investigations on use of NSOME to improve speech production revealed that only eight articles had sound methodology and went through a peer-reviewed process for publication (McCauley et al., 2009). The conclusions of this review revealed that there was insufficient evidence to support or refute use of NSOME. Our current knowledge on this topic is that the principles of EBP do not support use of nonspeech exercises to improve speech targets. After an extensive review of the topic of NSOME in children, Lof (2009) suggested that if clinicians want to improve speech, they should target actual speech tasks.

Prosody

Prosody includes stress, intonation, and rate/rhythm that influence speech. Targeting prosody to improve intelligibility often involves complex modification of loudness, pitch, and duration. In discussing prosody, we want to consider the impact on both intelligibility and naturalness of speech. Duffy (2019) states that naturalness reflects the "overall adequacy of prosody" (p. 406). Targeting prosody may improve intelligibility (Duffy, 2019) and naturalness (Patel, 2002) when speech disability is severe and in mild disability, naturalness can be improved by working on prosody (Yorkston et al., 2010).

Modifying Speech Rate

Slow rate is very common among speakers with dysarthria (Duffy, 2019). Some clients have a slow rate because they physically cannot speak faster, and others may have developed a compensatory strategy of using slow rate to be more intelligible (Clark, 2020). For these reasons, when working with clients, our goal is often to slow speech rate, rather than increase it (Clark, 2020). That may seem counterintuitive. If the client is already speaking at a noticeably slower rate, wouldn't we want to have them speak closer to a normal rate? The answer, in most cases, is no because intelligibility improves when rate is reduced in speakers with dysarthria (Yorkston & Beukelman, 1981; Yorkston et al., 1990). One study showed that nearly all speakers with dysarthria had improved intelligibility after reducing rate but that speakers with severe dysarthria had larger improvements in intelligibility (van Nuffelen et al., 2009). Many studies have examined rate in different dysarthria types, using various rate control strategies, making it difficult to separately report and compare each finding. These differences also result in mixed findings of rate modification having a positive impact on intelligibility because the speakers and methods used are so varied. Yorkston and colleagues (2007) completed a systematic review of research and concluded that many techniques can be used to modify rate and those changes can impact intelligibility. This review concluded that further research is needed to provide more clinical insight into how rate is modified and the impact on different severity levels of dysarthria. Experts in motor speech disorders suggest that the use of rate control improves intelligibility, finding that reducing speaking rate may be relatively easy for clients to achieve (Duffy, 2019; Swigert, 2010). Rate control can improve intelligibility in several ways. Using a slower rate allows the speaker to hit their articulatory targets, rather than causing them to undershoot and not produce sounds clearly (Tjaden & Wilding, 2004). Using a slower rate may allow the speaker to have better coordination between the subsystems (Swigert, 2010). Another benefit of using a slower rate is that listeners have more time to process and understand what is said (Hammen et al., 1994). Blanchet and Snyder (2010) provide a tutorial of techniques shown by studies to be useful in rate control.

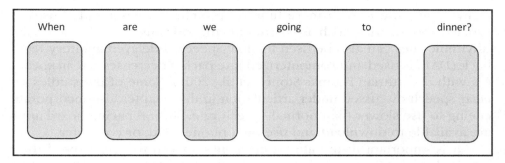

| When | are | we | going | to | dinner? |

Figure 5–1. Pacing board example.

To understand how to instruct our clients to modify their rate, it helps to know what people can do to slow their rate of speech. Speaking rate can be measured in articulation time and pause time, both of which are useful to listeners trying to understand a speaker (Miller et al., 1984). We can direct clients to reduce rate by explaining and modeling how to modify pause and articulation time (Logan et al., 2002). Articulation time can be increased if we instruct clients to elongate phonemes within syllables. When instructing clients to increase articulation time, discuss which sounds can be prolonged (vowels and some consonants, such as voiced fricatives, liquids, and glides) and those that cannot (stops sounds). Pause time is easier to modify than articulation time because pauses represent between 30% to 50% of total speaking time (Henderson et al., 1966). Pause time slows rate if the speaker uses more frequent and longer pauses between words. Clients who have reduced breath support may have short utterances and pauses that are not related to syntax or punctuation. This can affect intelligibility because listeners use pauses to separate the speech into syntactic units. If we take the pauses at places not related to syntax, for example, where a comma or period would be, speech is less intelligible (Hammen et al., 1994).

There are many strategies you can use to help clients slow their rate of speech. Rigid or metered rate control involves the client producing a one-word-at-a-time speaking style, usually involves a pacing technique and although the slowed rate may improve intelligibility, naturalness of speech is disrupted (Yorkston et al., 1990). Using a pacing board allows the speaker to say one word or syllable for each bar or circle on the pacing board (Figure 5–1). A similar strategy involves the client learning to tap the table without a board or tapping a finger or hand on their leg for each word or syllable spoken. A metronome can be helpful to help set the appropriate pace for your client. Another type of rate control involves the use of rhythm and is less disruptive to speech naturalness (Yorkston et al., 1990). Rhythm allows the speaker to maintain a more natural balance between pause time and articulation time. A rhythmic cueing task would involve the clinician pointing to words in a written paragraph using a rhythmic pattern, with more time on prominent words and pauses at syntactic boundaries, such as where punctuation calls for a natural break. Rhythmic cues can also be used to slow speech if delayed auditory feedback (DAF) is used and computerized rate pacing decreases rate in speakers with dysarthria (Thomas-Stonell et al., 2001). Some of the studies on clear speech discussed under articulation in this chapter also incorporate cueing to use slower than normal speech rate. Several pacing board apps are available to download and use on a phone, iPad, or computer.

It is important to monitor your client's speech to determine if their rate is slow and if there is a noticeable effect of rate on intelligibility. You should come up with a speaker-specific plan for what will benefit your client in the most functional manner. Changing rate of speech can be simple in therapy settings but requires cognitive functions to follow directions and recall how to modify speech (Clark, 2020). Swigert (2010) suggests considering if the client will be able to learn the technique and carry it over to functional everyday speaking situations.

Marking Stress Patterns

Stress occurs in speech when a syllable, word, or phrase is more prominent than others (Swigert, 2010). Lexical stress changes a word's meaning, so where the stress occurs determines the meaning. As an example, "Can you con**vert** this measurement to metric?" versus "She is a **con**vert to practicing a new religion." Speakers also use contrastive stress within phrases or sentences to alter their meaning. For example, in the sentence, "The **birds** ate the seeds," I will understand it was the birds that ate the seeds and not the squirrels. If the stress falls on the word "seeds," I know what the birds ate. Word intelligibility has been shown to improve through use of contrastive stress drills in adults with cerebral palsy (Connaghan & Patel, 2017).

There are workbooks and websites that contain contrastive stress drills; Swigert (2010) has many prosodic drill exercises in the DVD that accompanies her book. You can create your own stimuli, possibly related to the client's functional communication as well. Here is an example:

I wanted to invite you to dinner and a movie. (I am the one asking, not someone else)

I **wanted** to invite you to dinner and a movie. (This is what I'm asking you, not something else)

I wanted to **invite** you to dinner and a movie. (I'm inviting you, not just assuming you'll come)

I wanted to invite you to dinner **and** a movie. (Both dinner and a movie, not one or the other)

Clients may mark stress by changing duration of the word, pitch, or loudness but depending on their diagnosis, some of these may be easier for them to use. Swigert (2010) suggests listening to how the client attempts to mark signal stress and then improve on what they can do in other words and situations. Incorporating stress drills early in therapy may help improve the client's respiratory, articulatory, and resonatory abilities (Rosenbek & LaPointe, 1985).

Using Intonation

In speakers with no disorder, intonation affects intelligibility (Laures & Weismer, 1999). Speakers with disorders, such as dysarthria and AAOS, have impaired prosodic features, including intonation (Duffy, 2019). Addressing intonation in treatment may allow listeners to have a better understanding of our clients. Patel (2002) investigated speakers with dysarthria and found that some could use intonation to improve intelligibility with unfamiliar listeners. Speakers in this study contrasted questions versus statements using intonation changes.

At the word level, speakers combine stress and pitch to create intonation. Sikorski (2017) describes eight basic word level intonation patterns found in English. These patterns are detailed and examples are provided in Table 5–2. Swigert (2010) points out that there are minimal differences between the two three-syllable words where stress falls on the first

Table 5–2. Word-Level Intonation Patterns in English

Pattern Description	Examples	
One-syllable word with falling inflection	Ask	Huge
	Laugh	Saw
	These	Quite
Two-syllable words with stress on second syllable, falling at the end	Across	Believe
	Correct	Escape
	Itself	Progress
Two-syllable words with stress on the first syllable, second syllable unstressed	Bother	Coming
	Figure	Often
	Taken	Written

continues

Table 5–2. *continued*

Pattern Description	Examples	
Three-syllable words with stress on the middle syllable	Already	Appointment
	Beginning	Committee
	Discussion	September
Three-syllable words with stress on the first syllable, secondary stress on the third syllable	Alternate	Calculate
	Dynamite	Illustrate
	Patio	Recognize
Three-syllable words with stress on the first syllable, no stress on the other syllables	Avenue	Balcony
	Government	Medicine
	Regular	Theatre
Three-syllable words with primary stress falling at the end of the third syllable	Comprehend	Diagnose
	Guarantee	Introduce
	Overworked	Understand
Four-syllable words with stress on the third syllable	Definition	Isolation
	Macaroni	Observation
	Politician	Reputation

Note: Adapted with permission from M.E.E.C.: Intonation Patterns of American English, Lorna D. Sikorski, LDS & Associates. Print Edition, ISBN 978-1-883574-30-7—Workbook only (printed). E-Book Edition, ISBN 978-1-883574-28-4—Workbook only (E-book).

Table 5–3. Sentence-Level Intonation Patterns in English

Pattern Description	Examples
Lower pitch at the end of a statement of fact or opinion	She is a teacher at North High School.
Lower pitch at the end of "wh" questions	Who was at the door?
	What would you like for lunch?
	Where is your shoe?
Rising pitch at the end of questions with expected yes/no answers	Are you ready?
	Did he go to the store?
Falling pitch on last word in a list of items	His favorite pies are apple, pecan, and blueberry.
	They are traveling to England, France, and Germany.

Source: McKinney (2019).

syllable. Some clients may have difficulty differentiating some of these finer distinctions. Sentence level intonation may also be difficult for clients but providing information about question versus statement can be useful for the listener. Table 5–3 describes some of the most common sentence types and the typical intonation used. For resources related to intonation, look at materials for accent reduction, such as McKinney (2019), or Sikorski (2017). Another excellent resource with many lists of words and sentences can be found in Swigert (2010).

MANAGEMENT RELATED TO SPECIFIC COMMUNICATION DISORDERS

To this point, much of the discussion has been on the topic of subsystems of speech. This is commonly the way we treat individuals with dysarthria. In consideration of individuals who may experience reduced intelligibility due to voice disorders, the focus would be on respiration, phonation, and resonance. A thorough evaluation of the voice disorder will help determine which of the subsystems and specific tasks would be most helpful with each individual client.

Adult Apraxia of Speech

AAOS mainly impacts the subsystems of articulation and prosody. Some more severe clients may need treatment in the areas of respiration and phonation; with resonance being very rarely impacted (Duffy, 2019). Approaches aimed at improving intelligibility focus on reestablishing motor plans/programs which the client previously used during speech. Improving the ability to utilize these motor programs and set program parameters (e.g., speed) in specific situations is a desired target (Knock et al., 2000). These treatment approaches include articulatory-kinematic approaches, sensory cueing, rate and/or rhythm control, as well as combinations of these (Table 5–4). For a review of other treatment approaches related to AAOS, please see Duffy (2019) and Yorkston et al. (2010).

Head and Neck Cancer

It is challenging to adequately cover all areas related to improving intelligibility in clients with H&N cancer, as medical treatment and choice of speech options vary significantly. Results from formal intelligibility assessment should guide individualized therapy strategies and goals (Christensen & Dwyer, 1990). In considering subsystems management, clinicians must

Table 5–4. Summary of Management Approaches for AAOS

Approach	Description	Reference for Support and Details
Eight-step continuum (integral stimulation)	■ Imitation (watch, listen, and say it with me) ■ Multiple sensory models (visual, tactile, auditory) ■ Prompts and cues faded gradually as client's productions become more independent and functional	Deal & Florance (1978) Rosenbek et al. (1973)
Sound production treatment (SPT)	■ Techniques used include: modeling, integral stimulation, orthographic cueing, feedback ■ Stimuli based on the client's error patterns ■ Less cueing and modeling from clinician in first steps ■ Assistance provided when errors occur (contrast with eight-step continuum) ■ Flexible in stimuli and type of methods used ■ Simultaneous treatment of multiple sounds promotes generalization	Bailey et al. (2015) Wambaugh (2004) Wambaugh & Nessler (2004) Wambaugh et al. (2006)
Prompts for restructuring oral muscular phonetic targets (PROMPT)	■ Tactile cues supply pressure, kinesthetic, and proprioceptive information ■ SLP uses finger placements on the client's face and neck to show target positions for articulation ■ Considerable training is needed for SLP ■ Appropriate for clients where other methods have failed	Bose et al. (2001) Chumpelik (1984) Freed et al. (1997) Most studies are single-subject design, results are favorable, but evidence is partial.

Table 5–4. *continued*

Approach	Description	Reference for Support and Details
Motor learning guided treatment (MLG)	■ Practice of randomly organized functional words and phrases ■ Client pauses between words to judge response and make adjustments ■ Feedback provided by clinician after every 3rd production	Johnson et al. (2018) Lasker et al. (2008) Lasker et al. (2010) Case studies indicating need for further study to confirm positive results.
Script Training	■ Target phrases are chosen by client for functional communication situations ■ Phrases are practiced until fluent and client can use spontaneously in conversation ■ Scripts are used for practice of functional communication	Henry et al. (2018) Holland et al. (2002) Youmans et al. (2011)
Melodic intonation therapy (MIT)	■ Initially studied/used with clients with aphasia ■ Variation of singing based on melody, rhythm, stress ■ Client learns hand tapping (rhythm) and hums with clinician to add melody ■ SLP cues heavy initially but faded during progression ■ Helpful with clients with good verbal comprehension, non-fluent speech (Broca's aphasia)	Sparks et al. (1974) (aphasia) Sparks & Holland (1976) (aphasia) Zumbansen et al. (2014)

tailor treatment to medical and speech options available to each client. Targeting known error patterns and using compensatory strategies will create opportunities for more intelligible speech (Doyle et al., 1990). Clinicians should focus on management of appropriate subsystems for each client, recognizing that the needs for someone who has a diagnosis of oral cancer may be more focused on articulation, resonance, and prosody. Speakers who have undergone total laryngectomy have had their respiratory system decoupled or separated from their phonatory system. In these cases, we must address phonatory and articulatory challenges when working with clients using alaryngeal speech modes. These challenges will vary with the three types of alaryngeal speech. Speakers using electrolaryngeal speech (EL) need to find the optimal placement for the device and learn how to time turning on the device with speech onset. Esophageal speakers (ES) use different methods of injection and inhalation to produce various speech sounds. Training clients to use these methods can be difficult and may take time, as it requires careful adherence to a schedule where they meet criteria at one level before advancing to the next. Interested readers can find detailed descriptions of methods for instruction in esophageal speech in Graham (1997, 2005). Speakers using tracheoesophageal speech (TE) tend to voice all consonants, and voicing errors are the primary reason for reduced intelligibility in TE speakers (Doyle, 1988). One area showing promise was the finding that loudness and intelligibility improved in speakers using EL, ES, and TE when they used a heat moisture exchanger (HME) to help moisten and filter air that is inhaled through the stoma (Ackerstaff et al., 2003).

There are many client-specific considerations in working with this population and you will need resources to improve intelligibility with these clients. Readers are referred to the excellent resource by Doyle (2019) for specific information related to clients with H&N cancer. This book contains chapters related to specific modes of alaryngeal speech, as well as a chapter covering intelligibility following laryngectomy by Sleeth and Doyle (2019). The summary article by Graham (2006) has useful suggestions for working with alaryngeal speakers. Table 5–5 contains information related to alaryngeal speech methods focused on strategies to improve voicing and intelligibility based on Graham's summary. There are useful Internet resources related to alaryngeal speech, including information from the International Association of Laryngectomees (IAL) website found at https://www.theial.com.

USING OUTCOME MEASURES DURING MANAGEMENT

We can judge the success of our management by the outcomes we observe in our clients. For speakers with reduced intelligibility, we hope to see increased intelligibility along with functional communication that allows

Table 5–5. Management Approaches for Alaryngeal Speakers

Speech Modality	Description of Management Strategies Related to Voicing (consistency, quality, timing) and Intelligibility (articulation, rate, phrasing)
Electrolarynx	■ Optimal placement—use nondominant hand to place on same side neck or cheek, determine "sweet spot" by moving device to listen for best voice with least amount of noise. ■ Optimal placement for use with intraoral tube (if neck placement not possible)—use nondominant hand to place tube on same side in mouth at lower lip entrance to mouth (not in mouth). ■ Press "on" button of device with onset of production, release briefly at the end of phrases and press again to start the next phrase. ■ Practice short phrases as opposed to single words. ■ Articulate in front of a mirror for visual/auditory input. ■ Use distinct articulation (aka clear speech) with slightly slower rate—also assists with increased visual information.
Esophageal Speech	■ Practice for consistent voicing produced on command, using inhalation and injection methods. ■ Improve voice quality with air effectively vibrating the pharyngeoesophageal segment. ■ Develop quick and efficient intake of air for speech. ■ Use distinct articulation (clear speech) and practice voicing contrasts. ■ Start with reduced rate and increased loudness (clear speech,) but work toward more natural rate and phrasing. ■ Demonstrate appropriate loudness, intonation, and stress.
Tracheoesophageal Speech	■ Use valving of air using finger occlusion or a hands-free tracheostoma valve to completely occlude the stoma. ■ Practice using as normal a speaking rate as possible with pauses at natural points in conversation. ■ Practice voice and articulation, using increased length of utterance over time following success

Source: Graham (2006).

them to participate in the activities they enjoy. There are several reasons to complete further assessment to know the outcome of treatment goals. These measures can help us determine if treatment should be continued, changed, or discontinued. Insurance, Medicare, or other third-party payers may require documentation of progress. Clark (2020) suggests using this data to add clinical outcomes and knowledge in our field, which she describes as practice-based evidence. The way we take outcome measures may vary depending on the strategies and goals. Clark (2020) mentions two forms of outcome measures that align with the ICF classification system (World Health Organization, 2001). First, we can take measures of body structures and functions, such as number of breath groups or an inventory of speech sounds correctly produced. These types of assessment tasks were described in Chapter 3 as initial measures but can be used during management as outcome measures. Second, we can use functional assessment tasks, such as intelligibility measures and standardized measures of participation and quality of life, which are described in Chapters 3 and 4.

SUMMARY

When planning management for clients with reduced intelligibility, using frameworks to guide decision-making can be beneficial. These frameworks can direct your goals based on clients' abilities and areas in which functional communication will improve their quality of life. You should carefully consider which subsystems will have the most impact on your client's intelligibility and select targets in those areas. You can use information about the client's abilities and challenges gained through assessment to select goals that can improve intelligibility. Management of underlying issues related to the client's structures and functions for speech can improve intelligibility and allow for meaningful communication.

 # Case Study

Dysarthria Case: Christy considered Jack's prognosis, including the fact that he was making improvement in communication following his TBI. Her initial plan included management related to body functions and structures from the ICF (World Health Organization, 2001). Christy used principles of evidence-based practice and an interactive subsystem focus to develop

Jack's management plan. The plan included emphasis on respiration, phonation, and resonance initially with movement, to include articulation and prosody, using a bottom-up approach. Strategies for each subsystem were based on evaluation findings from the Perceptual Dysarthria Examination (PDE; Swigert, 2010) and included:

Respiration:

- PDE Rating—moderate
  - Short phrases secondary to reduced breath support
    - Christy instructed Jack in the use of diaphragmatic-abdominal breathing to increase his awareness of taking in maximum air for phonation.
    - Through an informal examination of Jack's breath groups, Christy determined that the optimal number of syllables for him to produce on one breath was six. She instructed him to practice taking breaths after six syllables, or sooner if needed. Christy instructed Jack's parents to cue him if he was not using optimal breath groups at home.
  - Reduced loudness
    - Using correct breathing and posture contributed to a slight change in Jack's loudness level.
    - Christy introduced Jack to an EMST device to assist him with increasing respiratory muscular support.
    - Jack learned to use an SPL meter to visualize when his voice was loud enough for different communication environments. Christy instructed him on how to judge loudness in different environments, including his classroom, home, and various social activities.

Phonation:

- ■ PDE Rating—mild
  - □ Reduced loudness
    - □ Christy knew from reading research that the methods she was using to improve respiration would likely assist with Jack's reduced loudness. He was referred to an ENT to determine if vocal fold closure was related to his accident. Results showed that vocal fold closure occurred, but with some level of weakness that would result in reduced loudness and breathiness.
  - □ Quality—breathy
    - □ Jack was instructed to time his phonation at the beginning of exhalation by practicing this breathing/speech pattern on vowels, then extending to words and sentences. This new pattern contributed to improvement in both voice quality and his ability to support longer utterances.
    - □ To ensure safe voice use, Christy instructed Jack how to practice vocal hygiene.

Resonation:

- ■ PDE Rating—moderate
  - □ Hypernasality
    - □ During Jack's visit to the ENT, the velopharyngeal port structures and movements were observed. Slightly reduced velar elevation was noted. The ENT recommended that Jack was a good candidate for a palatal lift and Christy assisted him in using this device during sessions.
    - □ A CPAP device was used during speech production to improve the function of muscles for velar elevation.

Articulation:

- PDE Rating—mild

    - Imprecise consonants

        - Christy set up intelligibility drills at the sentence level with Jack's best friend from college and his parents serving as listeners. She encouraged them to provide feedback to Jack, which allowed him to learn what they did not understand and for them all to practice breakdown and repair strategies.

        - Jack learned how to use "clear speech" by speaking to his listener as if they were hard of hearing. Christy encouraged him to use this technique often, especially in environments where he expected that listeners would not hear him well. In combination with the respiratory strategies, Jack could produce a louder voice when needed.

Prosody:

- PDE Rating—mild

    - Excess and equal stress

    - Flat intonation

        - Christy used prosodic exercises to assist Jack in using appropriate intonation. They used contrastive stress drills during treatment sessions, and Christy assisted Jack with generalizing by cueing him during conversational speech.

Christy worked closely with several individuals in Jack's life to cue him to use these strategies in his everyday life. His friend from college and his family members attended sessions to learn how to cue and repair communication breakdowns. Christy helped Jack make phone calls to his instructors to practice the techniques when she was with him. They completed some assignments to carry over speech strategies at the coffee shop, where he could practice ordering and interacting with others.

Case Study

Voice Disorders Case: Beth was motivated to improve and responded well during teletherapy sessions when Thomas guided her through a sample of the Phonation Resistance Training Exercises (PhoRTE; Ziegler & Hapner (2013). The intense exercises in this program increased in resistance and Thomas had read the evidence that PhoRTE can improve voice disorders in elderly clients with presbyphonia, as well as carryover to their conversational needs in life. Thomas had used PhoRTE successfully with other clients, both through face-to-face and teletherapy sessions. Based on the positive research findings, his previous clinical experiences, and Beth's interest in the program, he was confident that PhoRTE would be beneficial for her needs.

Sessions were scheduled once a week for an hour at a time when Beth knew her house would be free of family distractions, but her daughter would be available to assist with technology. During the initial session, Thomas discussed vocal hygiene with Beth with a focus on resting the voice (short voice naps) and consuming more water based on the report of reduced hydration. Thomas and Beth spent the first 15 minutes of each session addressing questions, briefly discussing how she incorporated vocal hygiene into her life, as well as review of home practice. The other 45 minutes were devoted to PhoRTE voice exercises. Thomas instructed Beth to keep her SPL meter 12 inches from her mouth so all readings would be consistent. Throughout all sessions, Thomas requested that Beth had water available, and he reminded her to take sips of water frequently. In the first session, Thomas asked Beth to read sentences containing all voiced sounds and they used her SPL meter to determine her average vocal intensity. This measure allowed Thomas to set her PhoRTE exercises at 50% to 60% of her vocal intensity range. Over the next three weeks, Thomas carefully guided Beth through the five PhoRTE exercises, so that she learned them well and was not straining her voice. At the end of each session, Beth was given written instructions for daily home practice and Thomas sent her an e-mail link to a video recording of himself demonstrating the exercises.

After five sessions, Thomas determined that Beth consistently produced the PhoRTE exercises at +20 dB above her habitual loudness (82 dB SPL). Thomas recorded Beth reading the CAPE-V sentences and rated her as a 10/100 (compared to 27/100 pretreatment). Thomas perceived little to no roughness and her loudness had perceptually increased. Beth completed a posttreatment VHI and obtained results that indicated normal voice function. Perhaps most importantly, Beth felt her quality and loudness had improved and reported not feeling strain or tension with normal everyday voice use. She had begun attending choir practice again and noticed that during social gatherings, she was no longer asked to repeat herself. As Thomas planned Beth's discharge from treatment, he provided her with a home maintenance program and encouraged her to continue PhoRTE exercises 3 to 5 times per week.

REFERENCES

Ackerstaff, A. H., Fuller, D., Irvin, M., MacCracken, E., Gaziano, J., & Stachowiak, L. (2003). Multicenter study assessing effects of heat and moisture exchanger use on respiratory symptoms and voice quality in laryngectomized individuals. *Otolaryngology-Head and Neck Surgery, 129*(6), 705–712. https://doi.org/10.1016/S0194-59980301595-X

Bailey, D. J., Eatchel, K., & Wambaugh, J. (2015). Sound production treatment: Synthesis and quantification of outcomes. *American Journal of Speech-Language Pathology,24*(4), S798–S814. https://doi.org/10.1044/2015_AJSLP-14-0127

Bane, M., Angadi, V., Dressler, E., Andreatta, R., & Stemple, J. (2019). Vocal function exercises for normal voice: The effects of varying dosage. *International Journal of Speech-Language Pathology, 21*(1), 37–45. https://doi.org/10.1080/17549507.2017.1373858

Barnes, J. (1977). *Voice therapy* [Paper presentation]. Southwestern Ohio Speech and Hearing Association Meeting, Cincinnati, OH.

Behrman, A., Cody, J., Elandary, S., Flom, P., & Chitnis, S. (2020). The effect of SPEAK OUT! and The LOUD Crowd on dysarthria due to Parkinson's disease. *American Journal of Speech-Language Pathology, 29*(3), 1448–1465. https://doi.org/10.1044/2020_AJSLP-19-00024

Behrman, A., Rutledge, J., Hembree, A., & Sheridan, S. (2008). Vocal hygiene education, voice production therapy, and the role of patient adherence: A treatment effectiveness study in women with phonotrauma. *Journal of Speech, Language, and Hearing Research, 51*(2), 350–366. https://doi.org/10.1044/1092-4388(2008/026)

Belsky, M. A., Shelly, S., Rothenberger, S. D., Ziegler, A., Hoffman, B., Hapner, E. R., . . . Gillespie, A. I. (2021). Phonation resistance training exercises (PhoRTE) with and without expiratory muscle strength training (EMST) for patients with presbyphonia: A noninferiority randomized clinical trial. *Journal of Voice*. Advance online publication. https://doi.org/10.1016/j.jvoice .2021.02.015

Beukelman, D. R., Fager, S., Ullman, C., Hanson, E., & Logemann, J. (2002). The impact of speech supplementation and clear speech on the intelligibility and speaking rate of people with traumatic brain injury. *Journal of Medical Speech-Language Pathology, 10*(4), 237–242.

Blanchet, P. G., & Snyder, G. J. (2010). Speech rate treatments for individuals with dysarthria: A tutorial. *Perceptual and Motor Skills, 110*(3), 965–982. https://doi.org/10.2466/PMS.110.3.965-982

Boone, D. R. (1997). *Is your voice telling on you: How to find and use your natural voice* (2nd ed.). Singular Publishing.

Boone, D. R., McFarlane, S. C., Von Berg, S. L., & Zraick, R. I. (2019). *The voice and voice therapy* (10th ed.). Pearson.

Bose, A., Square, P. A., Schlosser, R., & van Lieshout, P. (2001). Effects of PROMPT therapy on speech motor function in a person with aphasia and apraxia of speech. *Aphasiology, 15*(8), 767–785. https://doi.org/10 .1080/02687040143000186

Boutsen, F., Park, E., Dvorak, J., & Cid, C. (2018). Prosodic improvement in persons with Parkinson disease receiving SPEAK OUT!® voice therapy. *Folia Phoniatrica Et Logopaedica, 70*(2), 51–58. https://doi.org/10.1159/000488875

Bovo, R., Galceran, M., Petruccelli, J., & Hatzopoulos, S. (2007). Vocal problems among teachers: Evaluation of a preventive voice program. *Journal of Voice, 21*(6), 705–722. https://doi.org/10.1016/j.jvoice.2006.07.002

Bunton, K., & Weismer, G. (1994). Evaluation of a reiterant force-impulse task in the tongue. *Journal of Speech, Language, and Hearing Research, 37*(5), 1020–1031. https://doi.org/10.1044/jshr.3705.1020

Cahill, L. M., Turner, A. B., Stabler, P. A., Addis, P. E., Theodoros, D. G., & Murdoch, B. E. (2004). An evaluation of continuous positive airway pressure (CPAP) therapy in the treatment of hypernasality following traumatic brain injury: A report of 3 cases. *Journal of Head Trauma Rehabilitation, 19*(3), 241–253. https://doi.org/10.1097/00001199-200405000-00005

Cannito, M. P., Suiter, D. M., Beverly, D., Chorna, L., Wolf, T., & Pfeiffer, R. M. (2012). Sentence intelligibility before and after voice treatment in speakers with idiopathic Parkinson's disease. *Journal of Voice, 26*(2), 214–219. https://doi.org/10.1016/j.jvoice.2011.08.014

Chan, R. W. (1994). Does the voice improve with vocal hygiene education? A study of some instrumental measures in a group of kindergarten teachers. *Journal of Voice, 8*(3), 279–291. https://doi.org/10.1016/S0892 -1997(05)80300-5

Christensen, J. M., & Dwyer, P. E. (1990). Improving alaryngeal speech intelligibility. *Journal of Communication Disorders, 23*(6), 445–451. https://doi .org/10.1016/0021-9924(90)90030-3

Chumpelik, D. (1984). The PROMPT system of therapy: Theoretical framework and applications for developmental apraxia of speech. *Seminars in Speech and Language, 5*(2), 139–156. https://doi.org/10.1055/s-0028-1085172

Clark, H. M. (2003). Neuromuscular treatments for speech and swallowing: A tutorial. *American Journal of Speech-Language Pathology, 12*(4), 400–415. https://doi.org/10.1044/1058-0360(2003/086)

Clark, H. M. (2020, June 19). *Treating dysarthria in adults.* [Webinar]. American Speech-Language-Hearing Association. https://apps.asha.org/eweb/OLSDynamicPage.aspx?Webcode=olsdetails&title=Treating+Dysarthria+in+Adults

Colton, R. H., & Casper, J. K. (1996). *Understanding voice problems: A physiological perspective for diagnosis and treatment* (2nd ed.). Lippincott Williams & Wilkins.

Connaghan, K. P., & Patel, R. (2017). The impact of contrastive stress on vowel acoustics and intelligibility in dysarthria. *Journal of Speech, Language, and Hearing Research, 60*(1), 38–50. https://doi.org/10.1044/2016_JSLHR-S-15-0291

Dargin, T. C., DeLaunay, A., & Searl, J. (2016). Semioccluded vocal tract exercises: Changes in laryngeal and pharyngeal activity during stroboscopy. *Journal of Voice, 30*(3), 377.e1–377.e9. https://doi.org/10.1016/j.jvoice.2015.05.006

Deal, J. L., & Florance, C. L. (1978). Modification of the eight-step continuum for treatment of apraxia of speech in adults. *The Journal of Speech and Hearing Disorders, 43*(1), 89–95. https://doi.org/10.1044/jshd.4301.89

Doyle, P. C. (Ed.). (2019). *Clinical care and rehabilitation in head and neck cancer.* Springer. https://doi.org/10.1007/978-3-030-04702-3

Doyle, P. C., Danhauer, J. L., & Lucks Mendel, L. (1990). A sindscal analysis of perceptual features for consonants produced by esophageal and tracheoesophageal talkers. *Journal of Speech and Hearing Disorders, 55*(4), 756–760. https://doi.org/10.1044/jshd.5504.756

Doyle, P. C., Danhauer, J. L., & Reed, C. G. (1988). Listeners' perceptions of consonants produced by esophageal and tracheoesophageal talkers. *Journal of Speech and Hearing Disorders, 53*(4), 400–407. https://doi.org/10.1044/jshd.5304.400

Duffy, J. R. (2019). *Motor speech disorders: Substrates, differential diagnosis, and management* (4th ed.). Elsevier.

Duffy, O. M., & Hazlett, D. E. (2004). The impact of preventive voice care programs for training teachers: A longitudinal study. *Journal of Voice, 18*(1), 63–70. https://doi.org/10.1016/S0892-1997(03)00088-2

Dworkin, J. P. (1991). *Motor speech disorders: A treatment guide.* Mosby.

Evitts, P. M., Starmer, H., Teets, K., Montgomery, C., Calhoun, L., Schulze, A., . . . Adams, L. (2016). The impact of dysphonic voices on healthy listeners: Listener reaction times, speech intelligibility, and listener comprehension. *American Journal of Speech-Language Pathology, 25*(4), 561–575. https://doi.org/10.1044/2016_AJSLP-14-0183

Freed, D. B. (2020). *Motor speech disorders: Diagnosis and treatment* (3rd ed.). Plural Publishing.

Freed, D. B., Marshall, R. C., & Frazier, K. E. (1997). Long-term effectiveness of PROMPT treatment in a severely apractic-aphasic speaker. *Aphasiology*, *11*(4–5), 365–372. https://doi.org/10.1080/02687039708248477

Fulcher-Rood, K., Castilla-Earls, A., & Higginbotham, J. (2020). What does evidence-based practice mean to you? A follow-up study examining school-based speech-language pathologists' perspectives on evidence-based practice. *American Journal of Speech-Language Pathology*, *29*(2), 688–704. https://doi.org/10.1044/2019_AJSLP-19-00171

Gorman, S. (2000). Senile laryngis. In J. C. Stemple (Ed.), *Voice therapy: Clinical studies* (2nd ed., pp. 182–188). Singular Publishing.

Graham, M. S. (1997). *The clinician's guide to alaryngeal speech therapy*. Butterworth-Heinemann.

Graham, M. S. (2005). Taking it to the limits: Achieving proficient esophageal speech. In P. C. Doyle (Ed.), *Clinical care and rehabilitation in head and neck cancer* (pp. 379–430). Springer. https://doi.org/10.1007/978-3-030-04702-3

Graham, M. S. (2006). Strategies for excelling with alaryngeal speech methods. *Perspectives on Voice and Voice Disorders, 16*(2), 25–32. https://doi.org/10.1044/vvd16.2.25

Greenwell, T., & Walsh, B. (2021). Evidence-based practice in speech-language pathology: Where are we now? *American Journal of Speech-Language Pathology, 30*(1), 186–198. https://doi.org/10.1044/2020_AJSLP-20-00194

Gustafsson, J., Ternström, S., Södersten, M., & Schalling, E. (2016). Motor-learning-based adjustment of ambulatory feedback on vocal loudness for patients with Parkinson's disease. *Journal of Voice, 30*(4), 407–415. https://doi.org/10.1016/j.jvoice.2015.06.003

Hammen, V. L., Yorkston, K. M., & Minifie, F. D. (1994). Effects of temporal alterations on speech intelligibility in parkinsonian dysarthria. *Journal of Speech, Language, and Hearing Research, 37*(2), 244–253. https://doi.org/10.1044/jshr.3702.244

Henderson, A., Goldman-Eisler, F., & Skarbek, A. (1966). Sequential temporal patterns in spontaneous speech. *Language and Speech, 9*(4), 207–216. https://doi.org/10.1177%2F002383096600900402

Henry, M. L., Hubbard, H. I., Grasso, S. M., Mandelli, M. L., Wilson, S. M., Sathishkumar, M. T., . . . Gorno-Tempini, M. L.. (2018). Retraining speech production and fluency in non-fluent/agrammatic primary progressive aphasia. *Brain, 141*(6), 1799–1814. https://doi.org/10.1093/brain/awy101

Holland, A., Milman, L., Munoz, M., & Bays, G. (2002, June). *Scripts in the management of aphasia* [Paper presentation]. World Federation of Neurology Aphasia and Cognitive Disorders Section Meeting, Villefranche, France.

Huber, J., Stathopoulos, E., Sussman, J., Richardson, K., Matheron, D., & Snyder., S. (2019, September 23). Changes to speech production after Speech-Vive treatment in individuals with Parkinson's disease [Conference session abstract]. International Parkinson and Movement Disorder Society International Congress, West Lafayette, IN. https://www.mdsabstracts.org/abstract

/changes-to-speech-production-after-speechvive-treatment-in-individuals-with-parkinsons-disease/.

Hustad, K. C., & Weismer, G. (2007). A continuum of interventions for individuals with dysarthria: Compensatory and rehabilitative treatment approaches. In G. Weismer (Ed.), *Motor speech disorders: Essays for Ray Kent* (pp. 261–303). Plural Publishing.

Johnson, R. K., Lasker, J. P., Stierwalt, J., MacPherson, M. K., & LaPointe, L. L. (2018). Motor learning guided treatment for acquired apraxia of speech: A case study investigating factors that influence treatment outcomes. *Speech, Language and Hearing, 21*(8), 1–11. https://doi.org/10.1080/2050571X.2017.1388488

Kent, R. D. (2015). Nonspeech oral movements and oral motor disorders: A narrative review. *American Journal of Speech-Language Pathology, 24*(4), 763–789. https://doi.org/10.1044/2015_AJSLP-14-0179

Knock, T. R., Ballard, K. J., Robin, D. A., & Schmidt, R. A. (2000). Influence of order of stimulus presentation on speech motor learning: A principled approach to treatment for apraxia of speech. *Aphasiology, 14*(5–6), 653–668. https://doi.org/10.1080/026870300401379

Kuehn, D. P., Moon, J. B., & Folkins, J. W. (1993). Levator veli palatini muscle activity in relation to intranasal air pressure variation. *The Cleft Palate-Craniofacial Journal, 30*(4), 361–368. https://doi.org/10.1597%2F1545-1569_1993_030_0361_lvpmai_2.3.co_2

Kuehn, D. P., & Wachtel, J. M. (1994). CPAP therapy for treating hypernasality following closed head injury. In J. A. Till, K. M. Yorkston, & D. R. Beukelman (Eds.), *Motor speech disorders: Advances in assessment and treatment,* (pp. 207–212). Paul H. Brookes Publishing.

Laciuga, H., Rosenbek, J. C., Davenport, P. W., & Sapienza, C. M. (2014). Functional outcomes associated with expiratory muscle strength training: Narrative review. *Journal of Rehabilitation Research & Development, 51*(4), 535–546. https://doi.org/10.1682/jrrd.2013.03.0076

Lam, J., & Tjaden, K. (2016). Clear speech variants: An acoustic study in Parkinson's disease. *Journal of Speech, Language, and Hearing Research, 59*(4), 631–646. https://doi.org/10.1044/2015_JSLHR-S-15-0216

Lasker, J. P., Stierwalt, J. A., Hageman, C. F., & La Pointe, L. L. (2008). Using motor learning guided theory and augmentative and alternative communication to improve speech production in profound apraxia: A case example. *Journal of Medical Speech-Language Pathology, 16*(4), 225–231.

Lasker, J. P., Stierwalt, J. A., Spence, M., & Cavin-Root, C. (2010). Using webcam interactive technology to implement treatment for severe apraxia: A case example. *Journal of Medical Speech-Language Pathology, 18*(4), 71–76.

Laures, J. S., & Weismer, G. (1999). The effects of a flattened fundamental frequency on intelligibility at the sentence level. *Journal of Speech, Language, and Hearing Research, 42*(5), 1148–1156. https://doi.org/10.1044/jslhr.4205.1148

Liss, J. M., Kuehn, D. P., & Hinkle, K. P. (1994). Direct training of velopharyngeal musculature. *Journal of Medical Speech-Language Pathology, 2*(3), 243–251.

Lof, G. L. (2009, November). *Nonspeech oral motor exercises: An update on the controversy* [Conference session]. Annual convention of the American Speech-Language-Hearing Association, New Orleans, LA.

Lof, G. L., & Watson, M. M. (2008). A nationwide survey of nonspeech oral motor exercise use: Implications for evidence-based practice. *Language, Speech, and Hearing Services in Schools, 39*(3), 392–407. https://doi.org/10.1044/0161-1461(2008/037)

Logan, K. J., Roberts, R. R., Pretto, A. P., & Morey, M. J. (2002). Speaking slowly: Effects of four self-guided training approaches on adults' speech rate and naturalness. *American Journal of Speech-Language Pathology, 11*(2), 163–174. https://doi.org/10.1044/1058-0360(2002/016)

Mahler, L. A., Ramig, L. O., & Fox, C. (2015). Evidence-based treatment of voice and speech disorders in Parkinson disease. *Current Opinion in Otolaryngology & Head and Neck Surgery, 23*(3), 209–215. https://doi.org/10.1097/MOO.0000000000000151

McCauley, R. J., Strand E., Lof, G. L., Schooling, T., & Frymark, T. (2009). Evidence-based systematic review: Effects of nonspeech oral motor exercises on speech. *American Journal of Speech-Language Pathology, 18*(4), 343–360. https://doi.org/10.1044/1058-0360(2009/09-0006)

McKinney, R. (2019). *Here's how to do accent modification: A manual for speech-language pathologists*. Plural Publishing.

Miller, J. L., Green, K., & Schermer, T. M. (1984). A distinction between the effects of sentential speaking rate and semantic congruity on word identification. *Perception & Psychophysics, 36*, 329–337. https://doi.org/10.3758/BF03202785

Mullen, R. (2005). Survey tests member's understanding of evidence-based practice: A systematic approach to earmold selection. *The ASHA Leader, 10*(15), 4. https://doi.org/10.1044/leader.AN.10152005.4

Nacci, A., Fattori, B., Mancini, V., Panicucci, E., Ursino, F., Cartaino, F. M., & Berrettini, S. (2013). The use and role of the Ambulatory Phonation Monitor (APM) in voice assessment. *Acta Otorhinolaryngologica Italica, 33*(1), 49–55.

Netsell, R. W. (1998). Speech rehabilitation for individuals with unintelligible speech and dysarthria: The respiratory and velopharyngeal systems. *Journal of Medical Speech-Language Pathology, 6*(2), 107–110.

Pannbacker, M., & Hayes, S. (2008). Treatment for teachers with voice disorders: An evidence-based review. *EBP Briefs, 2*(6), 1–13.

Park, S., Theodoros, D., Finch, E., & Cardell, E. (2016). Be clear: A new intensive speech treatment for adults with nonprogressive dysarthria. *American Journal of Speech-Language Pathology, 25*(1), 97–110. https://doi.org/10.1044/2015_AJSLP-14-0113

Patel, R. (2002). Prosodic control in severe dysarthria: Preserved ability to mark the question-statement contrast. *Journal of Speech, Language, and Hearing Research, 45*(5), 858–870. https://doi.org/10.1044/1092-4388(2002/069)

Porcaro, C. K., Evitts, P. M., King, N., Hood, C., Campbell, E., White, L., & Veraguas, J. (2019). Effect of dysphonia and cognitive-perceptual listener strategies on speech intelligibility. *Journal of Voice, 34*(5), 806.e7–806.e18 https://doi.org/10.1016/j.jvoice.2019.03.013

Putnam, A. H., & Hixon, T. J. (1984). Respiratory kinematics in speakers with motor neuron disease. In M. R. McNeil, J. C. Rosenbek, & A. E. Aronson (Eds.), *The dysarthrias: Physiology, acoustics, perception, management* (pp. 37–67). College-Hill Press.

Ramig, L. O., Countryman, S., Thompson, L. L., & Horii, Y. (1995). Comparison of two forms of intensive speech treatment for Parkinson disease. *Journal of Speech, Language, and Hearing Research, 38*(6), 1232–1251. https://doi.org/10.1044/jshr.3806.1232

Rosenbek, J. C., & LaPointe, L. L. (1985). The dysarthrias: Description, diagnosis, and treatment. In D. F. Johns (Ed.), *Clinical management of neurogenic communicative disorders* (2nd ed., pp. 97–152). Little, Brown and Company.

Rosenbek, J. C., Lemme, M. L., Ahern, M. B., Harris, E. H., & Wertz, R. T. (1973). A treatment for apraxia of speech in adults. *Journal of Speech and Hearing Disorders, 38*(4), 462–472. https://doi.org/10.1044/jshd.3804.462

Roy, N., Gray, S. D., Simon, M., Dove, H., Corbin-Lewis, K., & Stemple, J. C. (2001). An evaluation of the effects of two treatment approaches for teachers with voice disorders: A prospective randomized clinical trial. *Journal of Speech, Language, and Hearing Research, 44*(2), 286–296. https://doi.org/10.1044/1092-4388(2001/023)

Sabol, J. W., Lee, L., & Stemple, J. C. (1995). The value of vocal function exercises in the practice regimen of singers. *Journal of Voice, 9*(1), 27–36. https://doi.org/10.1016/S0892-1997(05)80220-6

Sapienza, C. M., & Hoffman, B. (2022). *Voice disorders* (4th ed.). Plural Publishing.

Sapienza, C. M., & Troche, M. S. (2012). *Respiratory muscle strength training: Theory and practice.* Plural Publishing.

Sikorski, L. D. (2017). *Mastering effective English communication M.E.E.C.: Intonation patterns of American English* [eBook edition]. LDS & Associates. https://www.ldsassoc.com/m-e-e-c-mastering-effective-english-communication-complete-audio-series-e-edition/

Sleeth, L. E., & Doyle, P. C. (2019). Intelligibility in postlaryngectomy speech. In P. C. Doyle (Ed.), *Clinical care and rehabilitation in head and neck cancer* (pp. 231–246). Springer. https://doi.org/10.1007/978-3-030-04702-3

Sparks, R., Helm, N., & Albert, M. (1974). Aphasia rehabilitation resulting from melodic intonation therapy. *Cortex, 10*(4), 303–316. https://doi.org/10.1016/S0010-9452(74)80024-9

Sparks, R. W., & Holland, A. L. (1976). Method: Melodic intonation therapy for aphasia. *Journal of Speech and Hearing Disorders, 41*(3), 287–297. https://doi.org/10.1044/jshd.4103.287

Spencer, K. (2006). Evidence-based practice: Treatment of individuals with dysarthria. *Perspectives on Neurophysiology and Neurogenic Speech and Language Disorders, 16*(4) 13–19. https://doi.org/10.1044/nnsld16.4.13

Spencer, K. A., Yorkston, K. M., & Duffy, J. R. (2003). Behavioral management of respiratory/phonatory dysfunction from dysarthria: A flowchart for
guidance in clinical decision making. *Journal of Medical Speech-Language
Pathology, 11*(2), xxxix–lxi.

Stemple, J. C. (2011). *Vocal function exercises* [Film, educational DVD]. Plural
Publishing.

Stemple, J. C., Lee, L., D'Amico, B., & Pickup, B. (1994). Efficacy of vocal function exercises as a method of improving voice production. *Journal of Voice,
8*(3), 271–278. https://doi.org/10.1016/S0892-1997(05)80299-1

Stemple, J. C., Roy, N., & Klaben, B. K. (2014). *Clinical voice pathology: Theory
and management* (5th ed.). Plural Publishing.

Swigert, N. B. (2010). *The source for dysarthria* (2nd ed.). Pro-Ed.

Thomas, L. B., & Stemple, J. C. (2007). Voice therapy: Does science support
the art? *Communicative Disorders Review, 1*(1), 49–77.

Thomas-Stonell, N., Leeper, H. A., & Young, P. (2001). Evaluation of a computer-
based program for training speech rate with children and adolescents with
dysarthria. *Journal of Medical Speech-Language Pathology, 9*(1), 17–29.

Threats, T. (2007). Access for persons with neurogenic communication disorders: Influences of personal and environmental factors of the ICF. *Aphasiology, 21*(1), 67–80. https://doi.org/10.1080/02687030600798303

Tjaden, K., Richards, E., Kuo, C., Wilding, G., & Sussman, J. (2013). Acoustic
and perceptual consequences of clear and loud speech. *Folia Phoniatrica
et Logopaedica, 65*(4), 214–220. https://doi.org/10.1159/000355867

Tjaden, K., Sussman, J. E., & Wilding, G. E. (2014). Impact of clear, loud, and
slow speech on scaled intelligibility and speech severity in Parkinson's
disease and multiple sclerosis. *Journal of Speech, Language, and Hearing
Research, 57*(3), 779–792. https://doi.org/10.1044/2014_JSLHR-S-12-0372

Tjaden, K., & Wilding, G. E. (2004). Rate and loudness manipulations in dysarthria:
Acoustic and perceptual findings. *Journal of Speech, Language, and Hearing Research, 47*(4), 766–783. https://doi.org/10.1044/1092-4388(2004/058)

van Nuffelen, G., De Bodt, M., Wuyts, F., & Van de Heyning, P. (2009).
The effect of rate control on speech rate and intelligibility of dysarthric
speech. *Folia Phoniatrica et Logopaedica, 61*(2), 69–75. https://doi.org
/10.1159/000208805

Van Stan, J. H., Mehta, D. D., Petit, R. J., Sternad, D., Muise, J., Burns, J. A., &
Hillman, R. E. (2017). Integration of motor learning principles into real-time
ambulatory voice biofeedback and example implementation via a clinical
case study with vocal fold nodules. *American Journal of Speech-Language
Pathology, 26*(1), 1–10. https://doi.org/10.1044/2016_AJSLP-15-0187

Verdolini Abbott, K. (2008a). *Lessac-Madsen resonant voice therapy: Clinician
manual*. Plural Publishing.

Verdolini Abbott, K. (2008b). *Lessac-Madsen resonant voice therapy: Patient
manual*. Plural Publishing.

Verdolini Abbott, K. (Instructor). (2008c). *Lessac-Madsen resonant voice therapy* [Film, educational DVD]. Plural Publishing.

Wambaugh, J. L. (2004). Stimulus generalization effects of sound production treatment for apraxia of speech. *Journal of Medical Speech-Language Pathology, 12*(2), 77–97.

Wambaugh, J. L., Duffy, J. R., McNeil, M. R., Robin, D. A., & Rogers, M. A. (2006). Treatment guidelines for acquired apraxia of speech: Treatment descriptions and recommendations. *Journal of Medical Speech-Language Pathology, 14*(2), 35–66.

Wambaugh, J. L., & Nessler, C. (2004) Modification of sound production treatment for apraxia of speech: Acquisition and generalisation effects. *Aphasiology, 18*(5–7), 407–427, https://doi.org/10.1080/02687030444000165

Watterson, T. (2020). The use of nasometer and interpretation of nasalance scores. *Perspectives of the ASHA Special Interest Groups, 5*(1) 155–163. https://doi.org/10.1044/2019_PERSP-19-00029

World Health Organization. (2001). *International Classification of Functioning, Disability, and Health.* https://www.who.int/standards/classifications/international-classification-of-functioning-disability-and-health

Yiu, E. M., Lo, M. C., & Barrett, E. A. (2017). A systematic review of resonant voice therapy. *International Journal of Speech-Language Pathology, 19*(1), 17–29. https://doi.org/10.1080/17549507.2016.1226953

Yorkston, K. M., & Beukelman, D. R. (1981). Communication efficiency of dysarthric speakers as measured by sentence intelligibility and speaking rate. *The Journal of Speech and Hearing Disorders, 46*(3), 296–301. https://doi.org/10.1044/jshd.4603.296

Yorkston, K. M., Beukelman, D. R., Strand, E. A., & Hakel, M. (2010). *Management of motor speech disorders in children and adults* (3rd ed.). Pro-Ed.

Yorkston, K. M., Hakel, M., Beukelman, D., & Fager, S. (2007). Evidence for effectiveness of treatment of loudness, rate, or prosody in dysarthria: A systematic review. *Journal of Medical Speech-language Pathology, 15*(2), xi–xxxvi.

Yorkston, K. M., Hammen, V. L., Beukelman, D. R., & Traynor, C. D. (1990). The effect of rate control on the intelligibility and naturalness of dysarthric speech. *The Journal of Speech and Hearing Disorders, 55*(3), 550–560. https://doi.org/10.1044/jshd.5503.550

Yorkston, K. M., Spencer, K. A., Duffy, J. R., Beukelman, D. R., Golper, L. A., Miller, R., . . . Sullivan, M. (2001). Evidence-based practice guidelines for dysarthria: Management of velopharyngeal function. *Journal of Medical Speech-Language Pathology, 9*(4), 257–274.

Youmans, G., Youmans, S. R., & Hancock, A. B. (2011). Script training treatment for adults with apraxia of speech. *American Journal of Speech-Language Pathology, 20*(1), 23–37. https://doi.org/10.1044/1058-0360(2010/09-0085)

Ziegler, A., Dastolfo, C., Hersan, R., Rosen, C. A., & Gartner-Schmidt, J. (2014). Perceptions of voice therapy from patients diagnosed with primary muscle tension dysphonia and benign mid-membranous vocal fold lesions. *Journal of Voice, 28*(6), 742–752. https://doi.org/10.1016/j.jvoice.2014.02.007

Ziegler, A., & Hapner, E. R. (2013). The behavioral voice-lift. *The ASHA Leader, 18*(3). https://doi.org/10.1044/leader.FTR4.18032013.np

Ziegler, A., Verdolini Abbott, K., Johns, M., Klein, A., & Hapner, E. R. (2014). Preliminary data on two voice therapy interventions in the treatment of presbyphonia. *The Laryngoscope, 124*(8), 1869–1876. https://doi.org/10.1002/lary.24548

Zipoli, R. P., & Kennedy, M. (2005). Evidence-based practice among speech-language pathologists: Attitudes, utilization, and barriers. *American Journal of Speech-Language Pathology, 14*(3), 208–220. https://doi.org/10.1044/1058-0360(2005/021)

Zumbansen, A., Peretz, I., & Hébert, S. (2014). Melodic intonation therapy: Back to basics for future research. *Frontiers in Neurology, 5*, 1–11 https://doi.org/10.3389/fneur.2014.00007

CHAPTER 6

Speaker Management Strategies to Improve Intelligibility and Functional Communication

Key Points:

- ■ Clients can improve intelligibility using strategies for slow and clear speech.

- ■ The speaker's message can be altered to increase intelligibility by modifications such as using predictable, common words and including written cues and gestures.

- ■ Speakers can learn to use strategies such as getting the listener's attention before speaking and watching for signs that their message has been understood.

- ■ If face masks are worn, speakers should use more effort to use loud, clear speech to ensure they are better understood.

- ■ SLPs can bring their client's communication partners into therapy sessions to practice how to repair communication breakdowns.

Using the ICF model to plan treatment allows us to consider functional aspects related to each client's communication (World Health Organization, 2001). The previous chapter focuses on intervention aimed at the impairment level, as well as activity limitations. This chapter will continue with speaker-related strategies to improve activity limitations and participation restrictions. Activity and participation are related, however, activity refers to execution of tasks, and we define participation as involvement in life situations (Yorkston et al., 2010). Answering a question is an example of a task and returning a call to a friend represents participation. The perception of reduced intelligibility can lead to lower levels of communicative participation in functional life situations (McAuliffe et al., 2017). Clinicians can work together with their clients to plan treatment that will increase activity and participation by utilizing strategies to improve intelligibility.

Intelligibility and comprehensibility are related but should be clearly defined; allowing clinicians to understand how management planning can be accomplished in different ways to best meet the client's needs. Intelligibility involves what the listener understands from the acoustic signal (Duffy, 2019). Comprehensibility includes what Lindblom (1990) describes as "signal-complementary information." Comprehensibility allows the listener to take advantage of cues from the speaker, the message, and the way communication takes place. For a speaker with reduced intelligibility, listeners may need to rely on these cues that are not part of the acoustic signal.

It's critical to consider important differences between what we do when we measure intelligibility versus when we are working with a client to improve their intelligibility. We learned in earlier chapters that many factors can influence an intelligibility score. When we measure intelligibility, we try to control these factors, such as what the speaker says (e.g., word predictability) and how they say it (e.g., speech only, no visual cues or gestures). However, during management, we can use those aspects to the advantage of the speaker.

This chapter focuses on strategies that speakers can use to enhance what listeners understand. Strategies used to improve comprehensibility will improve intelligibility and vice versa. We can group these strategies into four categories, including speaker-related, message-related, communication-related strategies, and strategies that involve interaction between speaker and listener. The listener is an active communication partner who shares responsibility with the speaker for the exchange of information.

SPEECH-RELATED STRATEGIES

In an ideal world, the techniques discussed in Chapter 5, which focused on reducing or eliminating the impairment, would allow speakers to communicate effectively. Besides setting intervention goals focused on the impairment, speakers can use compensatory strategies and other interaction strategies to allow for active participation in communication. Speakers with reduced intelligibility can use strategies to help listeners get a better understanding of the spoken message. Clinicians should consider the abilities and challenges of clients when determining which strategies might be most useful. Clients who have moderately to severely reduced intelligibility may be the ones who need the extra signal-enhancing information, as opposed to someone with a mildly reduced intelligibility. Yorkston and her colleagues (1996) suggest that clients with language or other cognitive problems may not learn or generalize the strategies easily.

Slowing Speech Rate

Chapter 5 lays out the case for reducing rate of speech to increase intelligibility and various ways to help clients change rate. Clark (2019) suggests pausing between words, not separating syllables within words, including every syllable, as well as every word when using slow speech. She also suggests that maintaining intonation, which may require even slower speech, may be helpful.

Making Speech Clear

Using clear speech directions can help our clients with various speech disorders have increased intelligibility. Chapter 5 contains various directions for using clear speech and a summary of different clients that this strategy may assist. Tjaden and colleagues (2014) suggest directing your client to imagine speaking to someone who is hard of hearing, or someone who doesn't understand the language; this would mean to over-enunciate and speak clearly. Clinicians may find that different clients have more or less success with these directions, so change what works best for each client and their communicative partner.

MESSAGE-RELATED STRATEGIES

Speakers can modify messages in order to assist listeners in understanding the meaning. Chapter 4 introduces the idea that factors related to the message itself can influence intelligibility. In that chapter, we discussed measurement and how to control or keep those factors similar between measures. In management, we can think about the best ways to use the influence of those factors on intelligibility. We can now instruct the speaker how to change their message slightly to increase intelligibility.

Using the Most Effective Message Length and Type

Clinicians may want to select certain types of messages, based on factors related to the severity of a client's intelligibility. Speakers who have mild intelligibility impairment have higher intelligibility scores on sentences than on single words (Hustad, 2007; Yorkston & Beukelman, 1971, 1978). If you are working with a client with mild intelligibility impairment, listeners may use context cues from the other words in the sentence to figure out unintelligible words. Instructing your client to use complete, simple sentences may be the most effective type of message (Carter et al., 1996). Using shorter sentences increases speech intelligibility in adults with advanced dysarthria associated with amyotrophic lateral sclerosis (Allison et al., 2019).

Use of expected words and sentence structure can help listeners to greater understanding. Yorkston and colleagues (2010) suggest that clients avoid using telegraphic utterances to allow listeners' use of syntax to provide more information. For speakers with more severe dysarthria, letting the listener know what word class (noun, verb, adjective) may assist listener understanding (Beliveau et al., 1995). Clients can accomplish this verbally, in writing, or using a communication or alphabet board.

Choosing Predictable Messages

Predictable sentences result in higher intelligibility than those that are unpredictable (Boothroyd & Nittrouer, 1988; Duffy & Giolas, 1974; Garcia & Cannito, 1996a). This happens when listeners who do not understand what a speaker says may "fill in the blank" if a word or two are missing. Teaching our clients to use predictable words and sentences can assist listeners in correctly guessing at words they do not understand. Sentences that are related to each other result in higher intelligibility than unrelated sentences (Drager & Reichle, 2001; Hustad & Beukelman, 2002). Clinicians should instruct clients to keep sentences related to each other and not change topics without informing their communicative partner.

COMMUNICATION-RELATED STRATEGIES

Many useful strategies to improve intelligibility can enhance the communication experience provided by the speaker to the listener. The suggestions in this section align with comprehensibility because the extra information provided to the listener does not come directly from the acoustic signal of the speaker's words. Most of these strategies are common sense and some may work better than others, so it's a good idea to customize what you select for your client's needs and abilities.

Gaining Listener Attention Before Speaking

Listeners who are provided with both auditory signals and visualization of the speaker generally have higher intelligibility scores than those who are not given visual information (Barkmeier, 1988; Evitts et al., 2009; Evitts et al., 2016; Hunter et al., 1991; Hustad & Cahill, 2003; Keintz et al., 2007). Because listeners should be fully attending to understand a speaker with reduced intelligibility, gaining the listener's attention is a great place to start. A listener may miss important information and understand even less if they were not aware the speaker was going to talk. Alerting the listener to an upcoming message can enhance communication exchanges. Speakers can gain the listener's attention in several ways. Verbal signals might include, saying the listener's name, or "excuse me," or somehow indicating they are going to be sharing information. Nonverbal signals might include gently touching the listener, gesturing, or making eye contact. The speaker should be sure the listener is watching their face before speaking (Clark, 2019).

Setting Ground Rules for Communication

Our clients should learn to share strategies for how they want communication to occur (Duffy, 2019). Speakers and their communicative partners should establish a set of rules about how to proceed during communication and breakdowns in communication. This is a very personal choice, and a client may have different preferences for various listeners. Speakers should discuss with listeners how they want to be told if they are not understood. Rules to set might include how a listener will indicate if communication has broken down. For example, should the listener interrupt verbally, use a gesture, or wait until the speaker checks on comprehension? Some speakers may be comfortable having a listener interrupt midsentence whereas others may not. If both partners agree on the ground rules, breakdowns will be easier to identify and repair. For clients with severely reduced intelligibility, explaining that the goal is for the listener to get the meaning, but not necessarily to understand every word may be useful (Clark, 2019).

Providing the Topic of Conversation

Speakers with reduced intelligibility can provide information to listeners by letting them know the topic they will be discussing. We call this topic knowledge "semantic context" in research. Having semantic cues allows listeners to predict what the speaker might say and to rule out words that will not be expected. Categories are a useful way for a speaker to provide semantic cues to the listener. A speaker could point to the overhead menu in a movie theater before stating which snacks and drinks he or she might like to have. By indicating movie theater menu items, the listener can pay close attention to the expected words, such as "popcorn," "soda," or "candy." A verbal cue can be used if the speaker states, "I want to talk about tomorrow's weather." This cue can lead the listener to thinking about words related to weather, such as "storm," "snow," "sun." When the listener has the semantic topic cue of "weather," and if they are not sure if they heard the word "rain" or "train," then knowing the topic will help them make the right choice. Listeners provided with context report more positive attitudes towards speakers (Hustad & Gearhart, 2004).

There are different cues that could be used, depending on the needs of the speaker and listener. Speakers could provide spoken cues or write cues down. They can use pointing to word lists, pictures, calendars, or newspapers. Speakers can also point to or select items on a computer screen. Figure 6–1 provides an example of a board that could provide visual cues related to a topic, or overall speaker needs for listeners. Many researchers have examined the impact of topic cues on intelligibility and comprehensibility. Generally, these studies have shown that providing semantic cues, in addition to the spoken message, improves intelligibility

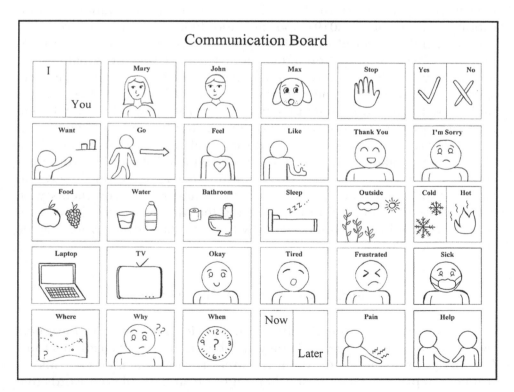

Figure 6–1. Communication board example. Illustrations by Claudia Torres.

and comprehensibility scores (Beukelman et al., 2002; Carter et al., 1996; Dongilli, 1994; Dowden, 1997; Hammen et al., 1991; Hustad & Beukelman, 2002; Utianski et al., 2011). As these studies showed improvement on single-word and sentence tasks for speakers with different etiologies and severity levels, topic cues may be useful for most clients. When speakers provide listeners with these types of cues, the use of these strategies will create the shared context described in Chapter 1.

Signaling Changes in Topic

Clinical experience has led Yorkston and her colleagues (2010) to conclude that the most common reason communication breaks down between partners who know each other well is due to changing topics without informing the other person. These authors suggest some speakers may need to provide the new topic whereas others may show a topic change, but not the specific topic, which might involve a gesture. Based on the strong research support for providing context, showing change and specifics about the new topic might be most effective. Speakers can signal topic shifts in many ways, including spoken, gestures, and written messages. Clinicians should select cues based on cognitive, pragmatic, and motor skills that are best suited to the client (Duffy, 2019).

Using Gestures to Provide Added Information

Gestures can provide listeners with information that is related, but not part of the actual speech signal. There are many terms and types of gestures, but we will focus on two types described by Garcia and Cobb (2000). Emblems convey meaning without a speech signal. If you are sitting across from your friend in a boring social situation, they may roll their eyes at you. The eye roll is a silent gesture, but you know that means your friend is also bored. Maybe your response is another emblem involving a quick head nod toward the door, silently showing your desire to leave. Your friend could nod their head or give you the thumbs up, both emblematic gestures conveying their message without words. Illustrators are movements that are related to the speech that help to visually illustrate the message (Yorkston et al., 2010). A client may choose to say "I'm thirsty" while using the gesture to drink, and this may have more success getting the message across with the visual illustration included. Placing your hands together next to your face and closing the eyes is a gesture that indicates someone wants to sleep. A hand up in front of you can signal, "stop." Your fingers can make motions to indicate movements such as cutting with a scissors or walking. There are many examples of gestures that nearly everyone understands. Therefore, a formal system, such as American Sign

Language, isn't needed. As long as the speaker and listener understand what gestures mean, communication can be enhanced. If you are interested in reading more about different types of gestures, see Ekman and Friesen (1972) and Garcia and Cobb (2000).

Gestures can be useful to our clients with reduced intelligibility in several ways. Studies of individuals with reduced intelligibility have revealed intelligibility increases with use of gestures (Garcia & Cannito, 1996a, 1996b). Interestingly, studies reveal that use of gestures may change the verbal message of the speaker. Cravotta and colleagues (2019) found utterances combined with gestures had higher fundamental frequency (perceived as pitch) and loudness than those without gestures. This means the gestures provide the listener with visual illustration, or signal-independent information, but are also providing listeners with useful acoustic information, such as increased loudness, which may improve intelligibility. Garcia and Cobb (2000) found that use of gestures increased the rate of speech in a group of speakers with dysarthria. Some people are just more naturally inclined to "talk with their hands" or gesture while speaking. For these individuals, incorporating gestures may come more easily, but most people can learn to use gestures to assist their listeners. Clinicians should determine if gestures are possible with clients, and determine if its use leads to improved intelligibility.

Providing Cues With Alphabet Supplementation

Speakers use alphabet supplementation when their speech is combined with a board containing alphabet cues (Figure 6–2). For individuals who need to spell out most, or every word, an alphabet board could serve as a low-tech augmentative device that would require more patience by the speaker and listener. Alphabet boards can provide a cue if the speaker points to the first letter of each word while vocalizing them. This provides signal-independent information through the phonetic cues. It also takes advantage of another strategy shown to improve intelligibility. If the speaker is using the alphabet board by pointing to letters, their rate will slow down. Hanson and colleagues (2004) systematically reviewed supplementary strategies and found six studies that examined 11 speakers' use of alphabet boards. Taken together, results indicated word intelligibility increased between 5% to 25%, and sentence intelligibility increased between 5% to 69% with the use of alphabet cues. It is interesting to note that speakers with more severe impairment showed greater levels of improvement and variability of intelligibility. Consider each client's needs and abilities for use of an alphabet board. Yorkston and colleagues (2010) describe advantages that include low cost, minimal training, usefulness in repairing communication breakdowns. Disadvantages included requirement of an external board, impact on rate and interaction with listener, and literacy levels needed for both communication partners.

A	B	C	D	Yes	No
E	F	G	H	Pain	Help
I	J	K	L	M	N
O	P	Q	R	S	T
U	V	W	X	Y	Z
Stop	Food	Drink	Now	Later	Restroom

Figure 6–2. Alphabet board example.

Watching for Signs of Listener Comprehension

We should teach our clients to maintain eye contact with listeners in order to monitor comprehension (Duffy, 2019). Speakers can also ask if the listener understood the message and determine which part the listener may have had difficulty with. A speaker who understands earlier in a conversation will have a better chance of using repair strategies to communicate. Waiting until the listener is completely lost or missing relevant information can cause more misunderstanding. Speakers can play a role in watching for signs of confusion or misunderstanding.

Scheduling Important Discussions

There may be times when a client knows in advance that an important conversation needs to take place. Setting up a time when both communicative partners can take part, free of distractions, will be helpful. The speaker may want to be sure that their energy level will be at its best and select an environment that will be quiet and well lit, allowing the listener the best access to acoustic and visual information.

Repairing Communication Breakdowns

If the listener doesn't understand the speaker, there is a communication breakdown. For any speaker, these breakdowns may occur more or less with different listeners or in various situations. A breakdown with a familiar partner may require different repair strategies than an unfamiliar partner (Yorkston et al., 2010). The level of familiarity, shared context, and topic knowledge will impact how these situations are handled. In speakers with reduced intelligibility, it may be useful for them to watch for signs or simply ask the listener if they understood. It is helpful if the communication partners have a predetermined way of handling breakdowns.

Strategies to repair breakdowns will often include repetition of the message that was not understood. Clark (2019) suggests if a listener indicates they did not understand, the speaker should repeat exactly as stated the first time. If repeating does not help, a new strategy might be better. After several repetitions, the speaker may want to rephrase what was stated. In this case, it would be a good idea to be sure the listener knows this by having the speaker verbalize or write that they will say it differently. Using another word with the same or similar meaning may provide success. Some clients can circumlocute or describe a word that a listener might not understand. If a speaker is talking about their "Aunt Tilly" but the listener does not understand, someone in the family might understand a description of "mother's sister." Someone not familiar with the speaker's family would need a different description. As you can see, these types of repairs will vary by many factors, so advanced planning, practice, and even role modeling with our clients can be helpful.

Incorporating All Useful Modalities

Duffy (2019) describes this as "establish what works best when" (p. 420). Combining strategies can be useful for many clients. One reason some of the research on intelligibility is complicated is that quite a few studies have examined use of more than one strategy. As one example, Tjaden and colleagues (2014) examined use of clear, loud, and slow speech in individuals with Parkinson's disease. Clients can use the strategies discussed in this chapter individually, but they may also work more effectively when combined. It will be helpful for your client if you determine which strategies work best with different listeners or environments, keeping in mind that combining strategies may be the best choice.

Considering the Impact of a Face Mask on Communication

Speakers who wear face masks are most likely providing less visual and auditory information to their listeners (Corey et al., 2020; Vos et al., 2021). In this instance, breakdowns may occur more often so more effort will be needed by our clients. We should counsel them to make an increased effort to produce loud, clear speech when wearing a mask. Checking whether listeners have understood will be a strategy that can help repair any breakdowns of information exchange. Speakers who must wear a face mask may want to provide written, alphabet supplementation, or other nonverbal cues to listeners to get their message across efficiently.

STRATEGIES SPECIFIC TO SPEAKERS WITH VOICE OR HEAD AND NECK CANCER

Most of the strategies suggested in this chapter will apply to clients who have reduced intelligibility related to voice or H&N cancer, although research on their effectiveness is tied to motor speech disorders. For specific training related to clients with H&N cancer, the book edited by Doyle (2019) will be a helpful resource. Nagle (2019) suggests that speakers using electrolaryngeal speech (EL) may have additional challenges using some strategies, such as when one hand is tied up holding the EL device. This may reduce the amount of signal-independent information available to listeners. If a speaker is relying on the oral-type EL device, there may be less visual speech information or unusual facial expressions or movements (Nagle, 2019). Some speakers using tracheoesophageal puncture (TEP) devices may need to cover the stoma or speaking valve with one hand, which could prevent use of gestures or motions with these clients as well. Clients who have had surgical treatment for H&N cancer may have anatomy or movements that are visually distracting to listeners. Clinicians working with these clients should consider the best use of strategies that the clients can use, realizing that the acoustic signal compromises intelligibility in many speakers with H&N cancer.

INTERVENTION OBJECTIVES TO BE FACILITATED BY THE CLINICIAN

As the SLP, you will introduce most of the strategies aimed at improving your client's intelligibility. You may work with the client on speaker strategies and subsystem management techniques. Clark (2019) suggests highlighting the value of the client being understood the first time so that repair strategies are not needed. The benefit of individual strategies will not be the same for each client. However, the value will also be different for the same client over time, depending on recovery or disease progression.

You can also bring in the client's communicative partners to learn listener strategies (Chapter 7) and the communicative process strategies, such as repairing breakdowns. Your client and their listeners should practice using the strategies and repairs so the process will flow smoothly when they are needed in real life. Teach your client and their family/caregivers that successful communication means effort by both the speaker and listener. These individuals should also share responsibility to ensure the environment is optimal for communication.

SUMMARY

Speakers with reduced intelligibility can use many strategies to improve communication effectiveness. Clinicians can use evidence from many investigations on these strategies. Relying on finding a study that lays out each client's exact situation may be frustrating because of the wide variation of study factors, such as speaker's medical diagnosis, disorder, and severity. There could also be confusion based on the speaker's task, which may include reading or speaking, and the types of strategies used. Whereas some studies examine one strategy, such as alphabet supplementation, others combine strategies and some measure comprehension, while others measure intelligibility. If you want to find research related to a client's specific dysarthria type or severity, the review provided by Hanson and colleagues (2004) is available through the Academy of Neurologic Communication Disorders and Sciences (ANCDS) website. Strategies described in this chapter were found to be useful with some speakers under certain conditions. It will be helpful for you to look at the suggestions and try some strategies with your client to see what seems most helpful. You may want to measure intelligibility or comprehension before and after, using certain strategies to conduct your own research for your client's specific needs. Keep in mind that additional information provided by strategies in this chapter will create a shared context between the speaker and their communicative partners.

Case Study

Dysarthria Case: Jack's use of clear speech was successful and was a good example of a strategy that he used to alter his own speech to improve intelligibility. Christy instructed Jack on how he could plan his message to be better understood by listeners. For example, they discussed that using complete, simple sentences would give his listeners context and improve his ability to use his breath control effectively. Christy also taught Jack strategies to help him adapt his communication skills. He learned that getting the listener's attention before speaking helps the listener to know to focus on his speech and watch his face and body for cues. Jack and his parents discussed a system of ground rules for the best ways and times for them to communicate about important topics. Jack learned it is important to provide the topic to his listeners and to let them know if he is going to change topics. During sessions in the clinic, and those held in Jack's real-world environment, Christy assisted Jack in using repair strategies when listeners did not understand him.

 # Case Study

Voice Disorders Case: Thomas encouraged Beth to use her supported respiration and louder voice without strain in all speaking situations, including when singing. They also practiced using these skills with a face mask as there were times she needed to wear one and be understood by unfamiliar listeners. They discussed the use of different types of masks, and how she needed to use increased effort to be loud and clear when wearing a mask. Thomas taught Beth how to signal topic changes and provide topics to listeners who may have more trouble hearing her, especially with her neighbor who wears a hearing aid. She practiced using gestures during the teletherapy sessions and how to check more often for listener comprehension of what she said.

REFERENCES

Allison, K. M., Yunusova, Y., & Green, J. R. (2019). Shorter sentence length maximizes intelligibility and speech motor performance in persons with dysarthria due to amyotrophic lateral sclerosis. *American Journal of Speech-Language Pathology, 28*(1), 96–107. https://doi.org/10.1044/2018_AJSLP-18-0049

Barkmeier, J. M. (1988). *Intelligibility of dysarthric speakers: Audio-only and audio-visual presentations.* [Master's thesis, University of Iowa]. Iowa Research Online. https://doi.org/10.17077/etd.dvdycbts

Beliveau, C., Hodge, M., & Hagler, P. (1995). Effective supplemental linguistic cues on the intelligibility of severely dysarthric speakers. *Augmentative and Alternative Communication, 11*(3), 176–186. https://doi.org/10.1080/07434619512331277299

Beukelman, D. R., Fager, S., Ullman, C., Hanson, E. K., & Logeman, J. A. (2002). The impact of speech supplementation and clear speech on the intelligibility and speaking rate of speakers with traumatic brain injury. *Journal of Medical Speech-Language Pathology, 10*(4), 237–242.

Boothroyd, A., & Nittrouer, S. (1988). Mathematical treatment of context effects in phoneme and word recognition. *The Journal of the Acoustical Society of America, 84*(1), 101–114. https://doi.org/10.1121/1.396976

Carter, C. R., Yorkston, K. M., Strand, E. A., & Hammen, V. L. (1996). The effect of semantic and syntactic content on the actual and estimated sentence intelligibility of dysarthric speakers. In D. A. Robin, K. M. Yorkston, & D. R. Beukelman (Eds.), *Disorders of motor speech: Assessment, treatment, and clinical characterization* (pp. 67–88). Brookes.

Clark, H. (2019, April 10). *Treatment of dysarthria in adults with acute, chronic, and degenerative conditions* [PowerPoint slides]. North Carolina Speech-Language and Hearing Association.

Corey, R. M., Jones, U., & Singer, A. C. (2020). Acoustic effects of medical, cloth, and transparent face masks on speech signals. *The Journal of the Acoustical Society of America, 148*(4), 2371–2375. https://doi.org/10.1121/10.0002279

Cravotta, A., Grazia Busà, M., & Prieto, P. (2019). Effects of encouraging the use of gestures on speech. *Journal of Speech, Language, and Hearing Research, 62*(9) 3204–3219. https://doi.org/10.1044/2019_JSLHR-S-18-0493

Dongilli, P. (1994). Semantic context and speech intelligibility. In J. A. Till, K. M. Yorkston, & D. R. Beukelman (Eds.), *Motor speech disorders: Advances in assessment and treatment* (pp. 175–192). Brookes.

Dowden, P. (1997) Augmentative and alternative communication decision making for children with severely unintelligible speech. *Augmentative and Alternative Communication, 13*(1), 48–59. https://doi.org/10.1080/07434619712331277838

Doyle, P. C. (Ed.). (2019). *Clinical care and rehabilitation in head and neck cancer.* Springer. https://doi.org/10.1007/978-3-030-04702-3

Drager, K. D., & Reichle, J. E. (2001). Effects of discourse context on the intelligibility of synthesized speech for young adult and older adult listeners: Applications for AAC. *Journal of Speech, Language, and Hearing Research, 44*(5), 1052–1057. https://doi.org/10.1044/1092-4388(2001/083)

Duffy, J. R. (2019). *Motor speech disorders: Substrates, differential diagnosis, and management* (4th ed.). Elsevier.

Duffy, J. R., & Giolas, T. G. (1974). Sentence intelligibility as a function of key word selection. *Journal of Speech and Hearing Research, 17*(4), 631–637. https://doi.org/10.1044/jshr.1704.631

Ekman, P., & Friesen, W. V. (1972). Hand movements. *Journal of Communication, 22*(4), 353–374. https://doi.org/10.1111/j.1460-2466.1972.tb00163.x

Evitts, P. M., Starmer, H., Teets, K., Montgomery, C., Calhoun, L., Schulze, A., . . . Adams, L. (2016). The impact of dysphonic voices on healthy listeners: Listener reaction times, speech intelligibility, and listener comprehension. *American Journal of Speech-Language Pathology, 25*(4), 561–575. https://doi.org/10.1044/2016_AJSLP-14-0183

Evitts, P. M., Van Dine, A., & Holler, A. (2009). Effects of audio-visual information and mode of speech on listener perceptions of alaryngeal speakers. *International Journal of Speech-Language Pathology, 11*(6), 450–460. https://doi.org/10.3109/17549500903003078

Garcia, J. M., & Cannito, M. P. (1996a). Influence of verbal and nonverbal context on sentence intelligibility of a speaker with dysarthria. *Journal of Speech, Language, and Hearing Research, 39*(4), 750–760. https://doi.org/10.1044/jshr.3904.750

Garcia, J. M., & Cannito, M. P. (1996b). Top down influences on the intelligibility of a dysarthric speaker: Addition of natural gestures and situational context. In D. A. Robin, K. M. Yorkston, & D. R. Beukelman (Eds.), *Disorders of motor speech: Assessment, treatment, and clinical characterization* (pp. 89–104). Brookes.

Garcia, J. M., & Cobb, D. S. (2000). The effects of gesturing on speech intelligibility and rate in ALS dysarthria: A case study. *Journal of Medical Speech-Language Pathology, 8*(4), 353–357.

Hammen, V. L., Yorkston, K. M., & Dowden, P. A. (1991). Index of contextual intelligibility I: Impact of semantic context in dysarthria. In C. A. Moore, K. M. Yorkston, & D. R. Beukelman (Eds.), *Dysarthria and apraxia of speech: Perspectives on intervention* (pp. 43–54). Brookes.

Hanson, E. K., Yorkston, K. M., & Beukelman, D. R. (2004). Speech supplementation techniques for dysarthria: A systematic review. *Journal of Medical Speech-Language Pathology, 12*(2), ix–xxix.

Hunter, L., Pring, T., & Martin, S. (1991). The use of strategies to increase speech intelligibility in cerebral palsy: An experimental evaluation. *International Journal of Language and Communication Disorders, 26*(2), 163–174. https://doi.org/10.3109/13682829109012001

Hustad, K. C. (2007). Effects of speech stimuli and dysarthria severity on intelligibility scores and listener confidence ratings for speakers with cerebral palsy. *Folia Phoniatrica et Logopaedica, 59*(6), 306–317. https://doi.org/10.1159/000108337

Hustad, K. C., & Beukelman, D. R. (2002). Listener comprehension of severely dysarthric speech: Effects of linguistic cues and stimulus cohesion. *Journal of Speech, Language, and Hearing Research, 45*(3), 545–558. https://doi.org/10.1044/1092-4388(2002/043)

Hustad, K. C., & Cahill, M. A. (2003). Effects of presentation mode and repeated familiarization on intelligibility of dysarthric speech. *American Journal of Speech-Language Pathology, 12*(2), 198–208. https://doi.org/10.1044/1058-0360(2003/066)

Hustad, K. C., & Gearhart, K. J. (2004). Listener attitudes toward individuals with cerebral palsy who use speech supplementation strategies. *American Journal of Speech-Language Pathology, 13*(2), 168–181. https://doi.org/10.1044/1058-0360(2004/017)

Keintz, C. K., Bunton, K., & Hoit, J. D. (2007). Influence of visual information on the intelligibility of dysarthric speech. *American Journal of Speech-Language Pathology, 16*(3), 222–234. https://doi.org/10.1044/1058-0360(2007/027)

Lindblom, B. (1990). On the communication process: Speaker-listener interaction and the development of speech. *Augmentative and Alternative Communication, 6*(4), 220–230. https://doi.org/10.1080/07434619012331275504

McAuliffe, M. J., Baylor, C. R., & Yorkston, K. M. (2017). Variables associated with communicative participation in Parkinson's disease and its relationship to measures of health-related quality-of-life. *International Journal of Speech-Language Pathology, 19*(4), 407–417. https://doi.org/10.1080/17549507.2016.1193900

Nagle, K. F. (2019). Elements of clinical training with the electrolarynx. In P. C. Doyle (Ed.), *Clinical care and rehabilitation in head and neck cancer* (pp. 129–143). Springer. https://doi.org/10.1007/978-3-030-04702-3_29

Tjaden, K., Sussman, J. E., & Wilding, G. E. (2014). Impact of clear, loud, and slow speech on scaled intelligibility and speech severity in Parkinson's disease and multiple sclerosis. *Journal of Speech, Language, and Hearing Research, 57*(3), 779–792. https://doi.org/10.1044/2014_JSLHR-S-12-0372

Utianski, R. L., Lansford, K. L., Liss, J. M., & Azuma, T. (2011). The effects of topic knowledge on intelligibility and lexical segmentation in hypokinetic and ataxic dysarthria. *Journal of Medical Speech-Language Pathology, 19*(4), 25–36.

Vos, T. G., Dillon, M. T., Buss, E., Rooth, M. A., Bucker, A. L., Dillon, S., . . . Dedmon, M. M. (2021), Influence of protective face coverings on the speech recognition of cochlear implant patients. *The Laryngoscope, 131*, E2038–E2043. https://doi.org/10.1002/lary.29447

World Health Organization. (2001). *International Classification of Functioning, Disability, and Health.* https://www.who.int/standards/classifications/international-classification-of-functioning-disability-and-health

Yorkston, K. M., & Beukelman, D. R. (1978). A comparison of techniques for measuring intelligibility of dysarthric speech. *Journal of Communication Disorders, 11*(6), 499–512. https://doi.org/10.1016/0021-9924(78)90024-2

Yorkston, K. M., & Beukelman, D. R. (1981). Communication efficiency of dysarthric speakers as measured by sentence intelligibility and speaking rate. *Journal of Speech and Hearing Disorders, 46*(3), 296–301. https://doi.org/10.1044/jshd.4603.296

Yorkston, K. M., Beukelman, D. R., Strand, E. A., & Hakel, M. (2010). *Management of motor speech disorders in children and adults* (3rd ed.). Pro-Ed.

Yorkston, K. M., Strand, E. A., & Kennedy, M. R. (1996). Comprehensibility of dysarthric speech: Implications for assessment and treatment planning. *American Journal of Speech-Language Pathology, 5*(1), 55–66. https://doi.org/10.1044/1058-0360.0501.55

APPENDIX 6–1

Checklist for Speaker Strategies to Maximize Functional Communication

Checklist for Speaker Strategies	
Speech-Related Strategies	☐ Slow Speech ☐ Clear Speech
Message-Related Strategies	☐ Appropriate Message Length ☐ Using Expected Words ☐ Selecting Common Sentence Structure ☐ Identifying Word Classes During Repair ☐ Keep Topics Related or Signal Topic Change

Communication-Related Strategies	☐ Agree on Rules to Address Communication Breakdowns
	  ☐ Verbal Interruption
	  ☐ Gesture to Signal Misunderstanding
	  ☐ Wait until speaker has finished, then inform of misunderstanding
	
	☐ Gain Listener's Attention Before Speaking
	  ☐ Spoken
	  ☐ Gesture
	  ☐ Touch
	
	☐ Ensure eye contact with the speaker
	
	☐ Use increased loud, clear speech effort if wearing a mask
	
	☐ Provide the topic for the listener
	  ☐ Spoken
	  ☐ Written
	  ☐ Pointing to object or picture

Checklist for Speaker Strategies (*continued*)	

	☐ Signal Topic Changes for Listener
	    ☐ Spoken
	    ☐ Written
	    ☐ Pointing to object or picture
	
	☐ Use gestures to supply extra information with speech
	
	☐ Utilize Alphabet Boards when needed
	
	☐ Check for listener comprehension
	
	☐ Schedule important discussions for ideal conditions
	
	☐ Use all modalities to repair breakdowns
	    ☐ Spoken
	    ☐ Written
	    ☐ Gestures
	    ☐ Alphabet Board

CHAPTER 7

Listener Strategies to Improve Intelligibility and Functional Communication

Key Points:

- SLPs can facilitate better communication if we work with both our clients and their communication partners.

- Variables related to listeners can affect intelligibility. These include age, cognitive abilities, effort, and familiarity with the speaker and their message.

- Listeners can be instructed to use strategies to improve communication, but will also develop approaches on their own for different types of speakers.

- Successful listeners use strategies such as using active listening skills, providing feedback, and using all available information from the speaker to understand the message.

The International Classification of Functioning, Disability, and Health (ICF) model (World Health Organization, 2001) allows clinicians to think outside the box of solely focusing on the subsystems producing speech and the reduced intelligibility that limits the activity of communication. Using this model guides us to further consider the most functional aspects of our client's participation in meaningful life situations. Yorkston and colleagues (2008) define communication participation as "taking part in life situations where knowledge, information, ideas, and feelings are exchanged" (p. 426). The focus of management should not be solely on the speakers, but should involve anyone who can affect the communication exchange.

Communication is a two-way street and involves both the speaker and listener's interactions. Olmstead and colleagues (2020) describe a process where the SLPs consider the speaker contributions, listener contributions, and the joint effort of both working together. The term "listener" is used throughout this book, yet not in the narrow sense of someone just hearing information. Our clients often need active listeners who are working to understand their message. A communication interaction allows us to see the efforts of both working together, not as individual efforts (Hustad & Weismer, 2007; Olmstead et al., 2020). Yorkston and colleagues (1996) suggest that shared responsibility can improve communication effectiveness. Communication partners, or listeners, may include family, friends, work colleagues, health care professionals, and others. It will be important for you to discuss this with your client, as each person's list of potential listeners will be unique and possibly evolving.

Weismer and Martin (1992) suggest that "Intelligibility is as much in the ear of the listener as it is in the mouth of the speaker." (p. 8). Our management should not focus only on the speaker's abilities to change and become easier to understand, especially when we are working with individuals who may not improve beyond a certain point. We can work with our client's communication partners to help them coordinate with the speaker to improve the sharing of messages. Listener strategies may involve changes in the way both the speaker and listener interact, and most are common sense ideas (Yorkston et al., 1996). Treatment is a partnership between speaker and listener that is facilitated by the clinician. The SLP can work with both communication partners to instruct them in using strategies in different situations. This chapter focuses on strategies that listeners can learn to adapt and use with speakers who have reduced intelligibility.

THE IMPORTANCE OF COLLABORATIVE EFFORTS

Health care is expanding into a greater emphasis on person and family-centered care, which provides even more support for including family, friends, and caregivers in the treatment of our clients with reduced intelligibility (Johnson et al., 2008). Person- and family-centered care involves joint effort into planning, delivery, and evaluation of clinical services. The mutual, beneficial partnership between clients, families, and clinicians is an important focus. Respect for the knowledge and experience that others bring to the table, as well as the consideration that each person's input is equally important, is a foundation for this treatment model (Baas, 2012). The ultimate goal of our management plan is likely to allow the client to share feelings and information with important people in their life. Participation by communication partners in a collaborative effort is critical.

Johnson and colleagues (2008) developed core concepts to facilitate effective person- and family-centered care. Using these concepts would be helpful when working with clients and their communication partners. Clinicians should provide an environment of respect by honoring the viewpoints and choices of the client and family. Incorporating their values, preferences, and cultural backgrounds into management allows the clinician to utilize both person- and family-centered care and critical elements of evidence-based practice. Providing accurate and useful information regarding the client's needs and skills can allow the client and family to take part in decisions regarding management at levels where they feel comfortable. Finally, a collaborative effort between clinician, client, and family should be used to determine the most useful strategies to improve intelligibility.

FACTORS RELATED TO LISTENER INCLUSION IN MANAGEMENT

When we incorporate listeners into our client's management, we want to remove some of the burden for the communication from the client. Their communication partner can take some of that responsibility. Intelligibility is, in part, based on the listener's contribution of taking in all information available in the speech signal, the speaker's message, and the communicative environment (Lindblom, 1990). Listeners use two types of information during the perception of speech (Liss, 2007). Recognition of isolated words involves no context, and we could think of this as similar to a word level intelligibility measure. The second is recognition of words in context, which is more similar to either sentence level intelligibility or comprehensibility. We can work with listeners on strategies to ensure they are taking in the most information during communication from all sources.

LISTENER VARIABILITY

Many years of research revealed that there are large variations among listeners during intelligibility tasks. Influences can include the type of disorder of the speaker and the task of the listener, including whether we ask them to transcribe or answer questions based on the speech sample. These variations are related to factors directly associated with the listener and may have a strong influence on results of intelligibility measures (Miller, 2013).

Listener Age

Investigators have examined listener age in studies that grouped listeners into two groups, with younger listener ages ranging from 18 to 30, and older listeners from 65 to 80 years of age. Some investigations have found that older listeners exhibit lower scores on intelligibility measures than younger listeners (Dagenais et al., 2011; Garcia & Hayden, 1999; Jones et al., 2004). Other studies have not found significant differences between these two groups (Dagenais et al., 1999; McAuliffe et al., 2013). One key factor to consider is that older listeners are more likely to experience hearing loss (Miller, 2013). As our clients may have older listeners as communicative partners, it would be smart to discuss this with them. Hearing evaluation and management to maximize listener hearing skills may be necessary for effective communication. Older listeners may need to know that they will need to use extra effort in these situations.

Listener Cognitive Abilities

Cognitive abilities of listeners, such as working memory (WM), can influence intelligibility scores. Park (2012) measured working memory in listeners who completed intelligibility transcription tasks and reported that listeners with lower WM capacity had lower intelligibility scores than those with higher WM capacity. This finding was stronger during sentence transcription, compared to single word transcription. Lee and colleagues (2014) conducted a similar study using words presented in background noise, adding even more challenge to the listeners' task. In this study, listeners with high WM transcribed more words correctly than those with lower WM. This research suggested that working memory skills can help keep the listener on topic. With sentences or even longer listening tasks, working memory may be needed to help the listener remember what the speaker said at the beginning of an utterance. Instruct your clients and their communicative partners to reduce cognitive interferences, such as competing background noises or distractions. Listeners who lack focus or have challenges with WM may need to use extra effort.

Perceived Listener Effort

During a communication exchange, listeners' limited cognitive resources are shared for various activities, including perception, attention, and memory (Kahneman, 1973). Completing a listening task with a communicative partner who has disordered speech, or is in a noisy environment, will require that the listener re-allocate cognitive resources in order to understand the message (Nagle & Eadie, 2018). When we work with our clients and their communicative partners, we should consider perceived listening effort (PLE), which gives us information about how taxing a listening situation is (Lemke & Besser, 2016). PLE can be measured through questionnaires or perceptual rating scales. For example, you could create a scale where "1" represents a listening situation with a professional announcer in a quiet room and "7" represents listening to a critically important message in a noisy environment (Beukelman et al., 2011). Studies have shown that PLE is higher when the listener is communicating with someone with various speech disorders, including ALS (Beukelman et al., 2011), Parkinson's disease (Chui & Neel, 2020; Miller et al., 2007), cerebral palsy (Landa et al., 2014), TE speech (Nagle & Eadie, 2012), and EL speech (Nagle & Eadie, 2018). Although these studies showed that reduced speech intelligibility was related to higher PLE, there was a wide variability of intelligibility scores. Listeners who reported higher effort during communication exchanges state that they felt like the extra effort lessened their personal connection with the speaker (Hirsch et al., 2021). There are some factors related to PLE that we cannot change (hearing status, WM). However, the use of strategies in this book can facilitate better listening conditions. If a speaker provides more information by using predictable messages and gestures, the listener may not need to use as much effort to understand what was said. Improving the communication environment may also increase intelligibility (Chapter 8). Ideally, the listener will realize that using strategies and improving the communicative environment results in the use of less PLE.

Listener Adaptability

Listeners adapt different strategies with various speech disorders, such as different dysarthria types (Klasner & Yorkston, 2005; Utianski et al., 2011). These findings have taught us that listeners are using active strategies in the moment when presented with different types of speech (Miller, 2013). Researchers attribute some of this variability to cognitive status, including attributes such as memory and attention (Lansford et al., 2011; Zekveld et al., 2012; Borrie et al., 2012a). These listeners modify their perceptual strategies when faced with disordered speech samples that vary from each other. The variability extends even among the same speakers with the same message (Garcia & Dagenais, 1998; Hustad & Cahill, 2003; Liss et al., 2002). Variability was noted among listeners rating electrolaryngeal speech (Nagle & Eadie, 2018). Like speakers, listeners will also bring their own unique skills to the communication event. This means that including the listeners in sessions to work with their speaker partners is even more important in facilitating the connection between the two. We can consider listener variability as their ability to adapt, which could be useful in implementation of strategies to be discussed later in this chapter.

Listener Experience With Speech Disorders

Listener experience is defined here as exposure to certain speech patterns or disorders as a whole, as opposed to listener familiarity, which describes contact with one particular speaker. This concept was described in Chapter 4, and is related to listeners involved in assessment. Borrie and colleagues (2017a) found that listeners who were exposed to one speaker could understand other speakers with similar speech disorders. A clinical use that takes advantage of this experienced listener might include listener training for health care professionals working with speaker populations, such as Parkinson's disease (Borrie et al., 2021). This training could lead to more effective communication between our clients and those who need to have a good understanding of their needs.

Listener Familiarization

The concepts of experience and familiarization are highly connected. In order to become a familiar listener, a person needs experience with a particular speaker. Familiarization involves exposing the listener to the speaker's message both through auditory and written modes. This means the listener hears the speaker reading sentences or paragraphs, and reads along with the written materials. Directions involve listeners paying close attention to both messages in order to understand the speaker. Many studies of speakers with dysarthria have revealed that familiarization with a speaker improves intelligibility scores (e.g., Borrie et al., 2012a; Borrie et al., 2013; Borrie & Schäfer 2015, 2017; D'Innocenzo et al., 2006; Lansford et al., 2016, Tjaden & Liss, 1995; Spitzer et al., 2000). Borrie and colleagues (2017) found that, although all listeners benefitted from familiarization, speakers with less intelligibility did not benefit as much as those with higher intelligibility. In a study examining effects of reading passage familiarization, Beukelman and Yorkston (1980) found that familiarization benefitted intelligibility the most for speakers with moderate intelligibility deficits. After familiarization, even SLPs experienced with speakers with dysarthria demonstrated higher intelligibility scores (Borrie et al., 2021).

If you plan to train listeners to become familiar with their communicative partners, findings from research can provide some clues about how to complete this. For example, using meaningful and functional materials or topics would be preferable (Borrie et al., 2012b). As listeners, we adapt to different speakers (dialects, voice qualities) and communication environments (noisy, no visual information) in our daily lives. For this reason, training listeners will probably not be a lengthy process; maintenance of intelligibility improvement may occur up to one month following just one familiarization training (Behn et al., 2021; Borrie & Schäfer, 2017; Kim & Nanney, 2014). When working with speakers with unpredictable errors, it may be difficult for listeners to learn the patterns they need to become familiar with (Borrie et al., 2018; Lansford et al., 2019, 2020). When determining if familiarization will be useful, consider the hearing ability, age, and cognitive skills of your listener (Borrie & Lansford, 2021). Using active training versus passive training can make a difference, with active leading to greater intelligibility gains (Borrie & Lansford, 2021). To use this active familiarization training, provide the listener with a written transcript of the intended speech targets (sentences or paragraph). Instruct the listener to carefully read along while listening to the speech sample. To work in the most functional manner, consider having both your client and their listener in the session to allow yourself to see how they each function individually, and also as a team. Borrie and Lansford (2021) provide a useful summary of how to train conversational partners.

COMMUNICATION ENTRAINMENT

When speakers and listeners adapt their communication style to become more similar to each other, this is called entrainment (Borrie & Liss, 2014). We have sound evidence that entrainment occurs in many communication parameters, both verbal and nonverbal (Borrie & Liss, 2014). Entrainment is less likely to happen when the speaker has disordered speech, such as dysarthria (Borrie & Schäfer, 2015). Table 7–1 contains examples of these parameters, along with references. Although there is some question about whether entrainment could have detrimental effects on intelligibility, entrainment may assist some speakers and listeners with improving intelligibility (Pickering & Garrod, 2004). Research is more focused on the types and reasons for entrainment, which will provide us with methods to consider in working with speaker/listener partners. For an interesting presentation by Stephanie Borrie, a researcher heavily involved in this topic, watch the Ted Talk listed here: (https://www.ted.com/talks/stephanie_borrie_entrainment_and_the_dance_of_conversation?language=en.) Borrie and colleagues (2019) provide methods for examining entrainment with speaker/listener dyads in clinical settings, which could be useful if you plan to address this directly this with your client.

Table 7–1. Communication Parameters Where Entrainment Has Been Noted

Communication Parameter	Reference
Speaking Rate	Giles et al. (1991)
	Local (2007)
	Street (1984)
	Webb (1969, 1972)
Pitch	Gregory (1990)
	Levitan et al. (2012)
	Local (2007)
Vocal Intensity (loudness)	Coulston et al. (2002)
	Local (2007)
	Natale (1975)
Voice Quality	Levitan & Hirschberg (2011)
	Neumann & Stack (2000)
Dialect	Giles (1973)
Phonological and Phonetic Features	Babel (2012)
	Pardo (2006)
Linguistic style	Danescu-Niculescu-Mizil et al. (2011)
	Niederhoffer & Pennebaker (2002)
Lexical choice	Brennan & Clark (1996)
	Garrod & Anderson (1987)
Syntactic structure	Branigan et al. (2000)
	Reitter et al. (2006)
Body Posture, Facial Expression and Gesture	Furuyama et al. (2005)
	Louwerse et al. (2012)
	Richardson et al. (2005)
	Shockley et al. (2003)
Respiration patterns	McFarland (2001)

Source: Borrie and Liss (2014).

LISTENER BARRIERS AND CATEGORIES OF STRATEGIES

Klasner and Yorkston (2005) investigated everyday (inexperienced, unfamiliar) listeners who were presented with samples of speakers with ALS and Huntington's disease (HD). After the listeners heard speakers, they were then asked about what they considered barriers to understanding. One barrier that was common to both speaker groups was that listeners could not understand words in sentences without context. From this, we reinforce the idea that we should encourage speakers to provide context and if they do not, listeners should ask questions to gain context. A second part of this study involved asking the listeners about strategies they used while listening to the speakers with dysarthria. These investigators grouped the reported strategies into one of four categories: cognitive, linguistic, segmental, and suprasegmental. Table 7–2 contains descriptions of

Table 7–2. Four Categories of Listener Strategies

Strategy	Definition	Example
Cognitive	Strategies related to cognitive processes including awareness, attention, and effort	■ Focusing strictly on the speaker and sentences to understand ■ Preparing to hear disordered speech
Linguistic	Strategies related to meaning or grammar	■ Using intelligible words to determine words that were not initially understood ■ Guessing or determining words not understood through context
Segmental	Strategies related to phonemes or phonetic structure	■ Putting pieces together into a whole ■ Using sounds to figure out words and words to determine sentences
Suprasegmental	Strategies related to rate, rhythm, or prosody	■ Breaking sentences down into individual words ■ Marking boundaries between words

Source: Klasner and Yorkston (2005).

those categories and strategies. Interested readers are referred to Klasner and Yorkston (2005) for additional information regarding development and use of the barrier scale. Results of this investigation showed that listeners used various forms of the strategies to understand the speakers. Listeners used segmental strategies more often with speakers with ALS, and suprasegmental strategies more often with speakers with HD.

Our take-home point is that listeners will use different strategies independently for themselves. It's a good idea to discuss with your client and their listeners what strategies work best. Johansson and colleagues (2020) interviewed speakers with Parkinson's disease and their communicative partners to determine changes in communication due to the disease. These investigators interviewed both partners, known as a dyad, together and separately. Interview questions focused on challenges to communication and what the partners felt contributed to communication success. Another important discussion included how the role of speaker and listener had changed since diagnosis. It's also important to know that strategies may change over time with disease progression (Depaul & Kent, 2000).

FUNCTIONAL LISTENER STRATEGIES

Bringing listeners into the therapy process can lighten the workload for speakers with reduced intelligibility. Listeners may come to the process with their own approach that helps them understand the message. However, there are some strategies that SLPs can teach them to improve communication. Ideally, the SLP can set up sessions to watch the communication partners practice using strategies so feedback and encouragement can be provided.

Using Active Listening Skills

Average listeners can think at a rate of about 500 words per minute, but a normal conversational pace of speech can range between 140 and 180 words per minute (McCoy et al., 2005). For some listeners, this may allow them more time to daydream or think about competing topics. For this reason, it is important for the listener to be actively involved with the speaker. This extra thinking and processing time can be used for listeners to take more information from speaker cues. SLPs can work with family members or caregivers to use active listening skills. It could be helpful to start with a simple discussion about keeping their focus on the speaker, watching for cues, and staying on topic. If the speaker is wearing a face mask, then the listener will need to use more effort than typically warranted and should also provide feedback if the message is not understood. Encouraging the speaker to use loud, clear speech may be helpful if a mask is contributing to a communication breakdown.

Watching for Signals That a Conversation Is Starting

If the listener hears the entire message and does not miss information at the beginning, understanding will be enhanced. It is important for the listener to be focused on the speaker, so watching for signs that the communicative partner is going to speak will be helpful.

Gaining Topic Knowledge

Listeners should find out from their communication partner what the topic of the conversation is. It is ideal if the speaker has learned to provide this information to listeners but, if not, the listener should directly ask. Communicative partners also need to be on the lookout for topic changes, which may be signaled by the speaker. If the listener feels the topic has changed but is not sure, they should question the speaker to find out.

Utilizing Visual Information

Communicative partners should be close together to allow the listener to see visual information, such as gestures, body language, and facial expressions. This information improves intelligibility for many speakers, and listeners should take advantage of it (Barkmeier, 1988; Evitts et al., 2009; Evitts et al., 2016; Hunter et al., 1991; Hustad & Cahill, 2003; Keintz et al., 2007). Being in another room or not visually focusing on the speaker will not benefit intelligibility. If the communicative partners are close together, the auditory signal will also be louder, which may improve understanding.

Using All Available Information

Written text, pictures, or alphabet cues allow listeners to have more information to supplement the spoken message. We should train speakers to provide information through various modes. SLPs can work with both partners together to help listeners learn to focus on all modalities.

Setting Yourself Up to Be the Best Listener You Can Be

Listeners may have challenges when taking in information provided by speakers. In the case of many of our clients, their spouses or caregivers may have visual or hearing difficulties. If the speaker is gesturing or pointing to pictures, the communicative partner needs to see them, so consequently, the partner's vision may need to be corrected with glasses or contact lenses. If the listener has a hearing impairment and the speaker has a speech disorder, the challenge for effective communication is increased. Audiological testing and the use of hearing aids, as needed, would be a benefit to communication in this situation. Listeners can improve their chances of understanding by maximizing their own communication abilities (Clark, 2019; Duffy, 2019).

Discussing Rules for Interaction With the Speaker

Listeners need to know how their partners want them to signal a breakdown in communication (Clark, 2019; Duffy, 2019). Teach both partners to communicate about how to address and resolve issues when intelligibility is reduced. Listeners can ask speakers to slow down and repeat words that were not understood. If listeners share what was not understood, it can help the speaker know what information they need to provide. If the speaker only has to repeat a word or phrase that was missed, it may be easier than restating the same sentence or thought (Schegloff et al., 1977). For example, "I heard you say you wanted to talk about a movie, but I didn't hear which one you wanted to tell me about." Avoid just saying "What?" and ask yes/no questions to provide clarification. Glossing is the practice of having the listener repeat each word the speaker says immediately after them (Clark, 2019). This can be useful in situations where the communication requires very high levels of feedback and monitoring. Glossing may be a useful strategy in combination with alphabet supplementation (Yorkston et al., 2004).

Providing Feedback and Encouragement

Feedback about the effectiveness of communication involves both speaker and listener responses. Both should monitor communication to determine if and when breakdowns occur. Providing feedback about what works and what doesn't will facilitate future communicative success. Listeners should also provide encouragement to keep their communicative partner from feeling frustrated when the communication is challenging (Duffy, 2019).

SPECIFIC STRATEGIES RELATED TO COMMUNICATING WITH INDIVIDUALS WITH VOICE OR HEAD AND NECK CANCER

Although the strategies mentioned throughout this chapter will also apply to listeners communicating with individuals with voice disorders, or alaryngeal speech, there are a few factors that are specific to these individuals we should consider.

Listener Strategies for Speakers With Dysphonia

Voice parameters, including quality and loudness, can reduce intelligibility (Evitts et al., 2016). Porcaro and colleagues (2020) investigated listener use of strategies for speakers with reduced intelligibility related to dysphonia. Strategies included (1) acknowledgment: providing a brief instruction to the listener that they would hear a voice disorder, (2) segmental: using other sounds in the word to decipher the word; (3) cognitive: paying close attention to the speaker and message; and (4) linguistic: using intelligible words to determine unintelligible words. The use of these strategies did not reach statistical significance to demonstrate an increase in intelligibility. However, use of the strategies resulted in clinical improvement in the study. Based on improved intelligibility in studies of speakers with dysarthria who use strategies, their use may produce functional improvement in speakers with dysphonia.

LISTENER STRATEGIES WITH SPEAKERS FOLLOWING HEAD AND NECK CANCER TREATMENT

If you are working with clients who use alaryngeal speech, many parameters related to voice and articulation will vary from non-disordered speakers. Following a laryngectomy or other surgeries, both audio and visual information related to speech may be altered. The presence of the stoma can be visually distracting to listeners (Evitts & Gallop, 2011). Surgical management may cause altered structures that can negatively influence visual information related to speech (Evitts, 2019). Listeners may be distracted by the presence of the electrolarynx.

Listener experience and familiarity can play an important role with your clients and their communicative partners. Several studies have shown that listeners who are experienced with TE speech will rate samples of TE speech higher than inexperienced listeners (Doyle et al., 1988; Finizia et al., 1998). As alaryngeal speakers may look and sound different from non-disordered speakers, listeners use greater effort and cognitive workload during communication exchanges (Alsius et al., 2005; Fraser et al., 2010).

Speakers who have had medical management of H&N cancer may provide significantly altered auditory and visual information during communication. Strategies previously described in this chapter will be particularly important with these clients. Listener perceptual training will probably be helpful with alaryngeal speakers. Allowing frequent listeners to practice with auditory and written transcripts as they work with their communicative partners helps reduce distractions, such as how the voice sounds or is produced, and the visual influences related to how the speaker looks or moves during speech.

EFFECT OF UNSUCCESSFUL COMMUNICATION ON SPEAKERS

This chapter focuses on the listener's contribution to successful communication, working along with the speaker. Baylor and colleagues (2011) completed interesting research focused on how speakers are affected by unsuccessful communication. The study involved speakers with seven different medical conditions, resulting in dysarthria, dysphonia, and the need for alaryngeal speech. Speakers responded with information about their feelings when challenges were encountered with communication. Some of the reported feelings included relying on friends and family for communication, or not feeling independent in public situations such as ordering in a restaurant or speaking to a doctor. These individuals felt others needed to be patient, giving them time to slow down or repeat as needed. Speakers also reported feeling as if others won't take time to listen or will wonder what is wrong with them, leaving them feeling vulnerable, embarrassed, or discouraged. SLPs who want to stimulate conversation between speakers and listeners could use discussion points from this study to allow an understanding of the impact of communication breakdowns occurring in the dyad (Baylor et al., 2011).

SUMMARY

Communication involves both a speaker and listener who work together as a team. There are factors that can influence a listener's ability to understand speakers with disorders, including listener age and familiarity with the speaker. Listeners, who have experience with different disordered speech, or particular speakers, will likely have increased understanding. SLPs can work together with speakers and listeners to facilitate use of listener strategies that may improve understanding. A checklist of listener strategies is included in Appendix 7–1. Listeners can take an active role in letting the speaker know specifically what was not understood. Working with both communicative partners to improve communication success may result in less frustration for both speakers and listeners.

Case Study

Dysarthria Case: Christy sat down with Jack early in the treatment process to discuss who his frequent communicative partners were. This list included his parents, sister, several friends from college, and his instructors. Christy arranged live or virtual meetings with each of these partners to instruct them of the importance of them working together with Jack on his communication. After these meetings, Jack's four instructors agreed to meet on their campus with Christy to go through familiarization training. Christy made a recording of Jack reading several paragraphs and brought that to their campus. The instructors viewed the video while reading the transcript to familiarize themselves with Jack's speech. During this session, Christy reviewed listener strategies, including using active listening skills. She focused on Jack's speech and his visual movements and provided feedback and encouragement to Jack. Friends of Jack joined one of his sessions by ZOOM (ZOOM Video Communications, Inc., 2020) to learn some of these strategies, and Christy included his family in his therapy sessions. They focused all strategies on the listeners seeing themselves as partners with Jack to increase his communicative effectiveness.

Case Study

Voice Disorders Case: Taking advantage of the fact that Beth's therapy was taking place in her home, Thomas occasionally set the session at a time when she could ask her family to be present. Beth interacted normally with her family during some of their session time while Thomas observed their communication styles and interactions. Thomas devoted a portion of one teletherapy session specifically to discuss listener strategies with Beth's daughter and husband. The group decided it was important to focus all attention on Beth when she was speaking to allow her to be heard without strain. They agreed that taking cues from her face, body, and the gestures she used were helpful as well. After minimal coaching, Beth, her husband, and daughter felt confident about providing feedback and using repair strategies if there was any lack of understanding. Beth mentioned she felt comfortable letting her friends from bridge club and from the church choir know she needs feedback if they do not understand her.

REFERENCES

Alsius, A., Navarra, J., Campbell, R., & Soto-Faraco, S. (2005). Audiovisual integration of speech falters under high attention demands. *Current Biology, 15*(9), 839–843. https://doi.org/10.1016/j.cub.2005.03.046

Baas, L. S. (2012). Patient- and family-centered care. *Heart & Lung, 41*(6), 534–535. https://doi.org/10.1016/j.hrtlng.2012.08.001

Babel, M. (2012). Evidence for phonetic and social selectivity in spontaneous phonetic imitation. *Journal of Phonetics, 40*(1), 177–189. https://doi.org/10.1016/j.wocn.2011.09.001

Barkmeier, J. M. (1988). *Intelligibility of dysarthric speakers: Audio-only and audio-visual presentations.* [Master's thesis, University of Iowa]. Iowa Research Online. https://doi.org/10.17077/etd.dvdycbts

Baylor, C., Burns, M., Eadie, T., Britton, D., & Yorkston, K. (2011). A qualitative study of interference with communicative participation across communication disorders in adults. *American Journal of Speech-Language Pathology, 20*(4), 269–287. https://doi.org/10.1044/1058-0360(2011/10-0084)

Behn, N., Francis, J., Togher, L., Hatch, E., Moss, B., & Hilari, K. (2021). Description and effectiveness of communication partner training in TBI: A systematic review. *Journal of Head Trauma Rehabilitation, 36*(1), 56–71. https://doi.org/10.1097/HTR.0000000000000580

Beukelman, D. R., Childes, J., Carrell, T., Funk, T., Ball, L. J., & Pattee, G. L. (2011). Perceived attention allocation of listeners who transcribe the speech of speakers with amyotrophic lateral sclerosis. *Speech Communication, 53*(6), 801–806. https://doi.org/10.1016/j.specom.2010.12.005

Beukelman, D. R., & Yorkston, K. M. (1980). Influence of passage familiarity on intelligibility estimates of dysarthric speech. *Journal of Communication Disorders, 13*(1), 33–41. https://doi.org/10.1016/0021-9924(80)90019-2

Borrie, S. A., Barrett, T. S., Willi, M. M., & Berisha, V. (2019). Syncing up for a good conversation: A clinically meaningful methodology for capturing conversational entrainment in the speech domain. *Journal of Speech,*

Language, and Hearing Research, *62*(2), 283–296. https://doi.org/10 .1044/2018_jslhr-s-18-0210

Borrie, S. A., & Lansford, K. L. (2021). A perceptual learning approach for dysarthria remediation: An updated review. *Journal of Speech, Language, and Hearing Research*, *64*(8), 3060–3073. https://doi.org/10.1044/2021_JSLHR-21-00012

Borrie, S. A., Lansford, K. L., & Barrett, T. S. (2017). Generalized adaptation to dysarthric speech. *Journal of Speech, Language, and Hearing Research*, *60*(11), 3110–3117. https://doi.org/10.1044/2017_JSLHR-S-17-0127

Borrie, S. A., Lansford, K. L., & Barrett, T. S. (2018). Understanding dysrhythmic speech: When rhythm does not matter and learning does not happen. *The Journal of the Acoustical Society of America*, *143*(5), EL379–EL385. https:// doi.org/10.1121/1.5037620

Borrie, S. A., Lansford, K. L., & Barrett, T. S. (2021). A clinical advantage: Experience informs recognition and adaptation to a novel talker with dysarthria. *Journal of Speech, Language, and Hearing Research*, *64*(5), 1503–1514. https://doi.org/10.1044/2021_JSLHR-20-00663

Borrie, S. A., & Liss, J. M. (2014). Rhythm as a coordinating device: Entrainment with disordered speech. *Journal of Speech, Language, and Hearing research*, *57*(3), 815–824. https://doi.org/10.1044/2014_JSLHR-S-13-0149

Borrie, S. A., McAuliffe, M. J., & Liss, J. M. (2012a). Perceptual learning of dysarthric speech: A review of experimental studies. *Journal of Speech, Language, and Hearing Research*, *55*(1), 290–305. https://doi.org/10.1044 /1092-4388(2011/10-0349)

Borrie, S. A., McAuliffe, M., Liss, J. M., Kirk, C., O'Beirne, G., & Anderson, T. (2012b). Familiarisation conditions and the mechanisms that underlie improved recognition of dysarthric speech. *Language and Cognitive Processes*, *27*(7–8), 1039–1055. https://doi.org/10.1080/01690965.2011.610596

Borrie, S. A., McAuliffe, M. J., Liss, J. M., O'Beirne, G. A., & Anderson, T. (2013). The role of linguistic and indexical information in improved recognition of dysarthric speech. *The Journal of the Acoustical Society of America*, *133*(1), 474–482. https://doi.org/10.1121/1.4770239

Borrie, S. A., & Schäfer, M. C. (2015). The role of somatosensory information in speech perception: Imitation improves recognition of disordered speech. *Journal of Speech, Language, and Hearing Research*, *58*(6), 1708–1716. https://doi.org/10.1044/2015_JSLHR-S-15-0163

Borrie, S. A., & Schäfer, M. C. (2017). Effects of lexical and somatosensory feedback on long-term improvements in intelligibility of dysarthric speech. *Journal of Speech, Language, and Hearing Research*, *60*(8), 2151–2158. https://doi.org/10.1044/2017_JSLHR-S-16-0411

Branigan, H. P., Pickering, M. J., & Cleland, A. A. (2000). Syntactic coordination in dialogue. *Cognition*, *74*(2), B13–B25. https://doi.org/10.1016 /S0010-0277(99)00081-5

Brennan, S. E., & Clark, H. H. (1996). Conceptual pacts and lexical choice in conversation. *Journal of Experimental Psychology: Learning, Memory, and Cognition*, *22*(6), 1482–1493. https://doi.org/10.1037/0278-7393.22.6.1482

Chiu, Y. -F., & Neel, A. (2020). Predicting intelligibility deficits in Parkinson's disease with perceptual speech ratings. *Journal of Speech, Language, and Hearing Research, 63*(2), 433–443. https://doi.org/10.1044/2019_JSLHR-19-00134

Clark, H. (2019, April 10). *Treatment of dysarthria in adults with acute, chronic, and degenerative conditions* [PowerPoint slides]. North Carolina Speech-Language and Hearing Association.

Coulston, R., Oviatt, S. L., & Darves, C. (2002). Amplitude convergence in children's conversational speech with animated personas. In *Proceedings of the Seventh International Conference on Spoken Language Processing, 4*, 2689–2692.

Dagenais, P. A., Adlington, L. M., & Evans, K. J. (2011). Intelligibility, comprehensibility, and acceptability of dysarthric speech by older and younger listeners. *Journal of Medical Speech-Language Pathology, 19*(4), 37–48.

Dagenais, P. A., Watts, C. R., Turnage, L. M., & Kennedy, S. (1999). Intelligibility and acceptability of moderately dysarthric speech by three types of listeners. *Journal of Medical Speech-Language Pathology, 7*(2), 91–96.

Danescu-Niculescu-Mizil, C., Gamon, M., & Dumais, S. (2011). Mark my words! Linguistic style accommodation in social media. In *Proceedings of the 20th International Conference on World Wide Web* (pp. 745–754). https://doi.org/10.1145/1963405.1963509

DePaul, R., & Kent, R. D. (2000). A longitudinal case study of ALS: Effects of listener familiarity and proficiency on intelligibility judgments. *American Journal of Speech-Language Pathology, 9*(3), 230–240. https://doi.org/10.1044/1058-0360.0903.230

D'Innocenzo, J., Tjaden, K., & Greenman, G. (2006). Intelligibility in dysarthria: Effects of listener familiarity and speaking condition. *Clinical Linguistics & Phonetics, 20*(9), 659–675. https://doi.org/10.1080/02699200500224272

Doyle, P. C., Danhauer, J. L., & Reed, C. G. (1988). Listeners' perceptions of consonants produced by esophageal and tracheosophageal talkers. *Journal of Speech and Hearing Disorders, 53*(4), 400–407. https://doi.org/10.1044/jshd.5304.400

Duffy, J. R. (2019). *Motor speech disorders: Substrates, differential diagnosis, and management* (4th ed.). Elsevier.

Evitts, P. M. (2019). The impact of postlaryngectomy audiovisual changes on verbal communication. In P. C. Doyle, (Ed.), *Clinical care and rehabilitation in head and neck cancer* (pp. 463–481). Springer. https://doi.org/10.1007/978-3-030-04702-3_28

Evitts, P. M., & Gallop, R. (2011). Objective eye-gaze behavior during face-to-face communication with proficient alaryngeal speakers: A preliminary study. *International Journal of Language and Communication Disorders, 46*(5), 535–549. https://doi.org/10.1111/j.1460-6984.2011.00005.x

Evitts, P. M., Starmer, H., Teets, K., Montgomery, C., Calhoun, L., Schulze, A., . . . Adams, L. (2016). The impact of dysphonic voices on healthy listeners: Listener reaction times, speech intelligibility, and listener comprehension. *American Journal of Speech-Language Pathology, 25*(4), 561–575. https://doi.org/10.1044/2016_AJSLP-14-0183

Evitts, P. M., Van Dine, A., & Holler, A. (2009). Effects of audio-visual information and mode of speech on listener perceptions of alaryngeal speakers. *International Journal of Speech-Language Pathology, 11*(6), 450–460. https://doi.org/10.3109/17549500903003078

Finizia, C., Lindström, J., & Dotevall, H. (1998). Intelligibility and perceptual ratings after treatment for laryngeal cancer: Laryngectomy vs. radiotherapy. *Laryngoscope, 108*(1), 138–143. https://doi.org/10.1097/00005537-199801000-00027

Fraser, S., Gagné, J-.P., Alepins, M., & Dubois, P. (2010). Evaluating the effort expended to understand speech in noise using a dual-task paradigm: The effects of providing visual cues. *Journal of Speech, Language, and Hearing Research, 53*(1), 18–33. https://doi.org/10.1044/1092-4388(2009/08-0140)

Furuyama, N., Hayashi, K., & Mishima, H. (2005). Interpersonal coordination among articulations, gesticulations, and breathing movements: A case of articulation of /a/ and flexion of the wrist. In H. Heft & K. L. Marsh (Eds.), *Studies in perception and action VIII* (pp. 45–48). Psychology Press.

Garcia, J. M., & Dagenais, P. A. (1998). Dysarthric sentence intelligibility: Contribution of iconic gestures and message predictiveness. *Journal of Speech, Language, and Hearing Research, 41*(6), 1282–1293. https://doi.org/10.1044/jslhr.4106.1282

Garcia, J. M., & Hayden, M. (1999). Young and older listener understanding of a person with severe dysarthria. *Journal of Medical Speech-Language Pathology, 7*, 109–112.

Garrod, S., & Anderson, A. (1987). Saying what you mean in dialogue: A study in conceptual and semantic co-ordination. *Cognition, 27*(2), 181–218. https://doi.org/10.1016/0010-0277(87)90018-7

Giles, H. (1973). Accent mobility: A model and some data. *Anthropological Linguistics, 15*(2), 87–105.

Giles, H., Coupland, J., & Coupland, N. (1991). Accommodation theory: Communication, context, and consequences. In H. Giles, J. Coupland, & N. Coupland (Eds.), *Contexts of accommodation: Development in applied sociolinguistics* (pp. 1–68). Cambridge University Press. https://doi.org/10.1017/CBO9780511663673

Gregory, S. W. (1990). Analysis of fundamental frequency reveals covariation in interview partners' speech. *Journal of Nonverbal Behavior, 14*(4), 237–251. https://doi.org/10.1007/BF00989318

Hirsch, M., Theirrein, M., Borrie, S., & Lansford, K. (2021, November 18–20). *Listener comfort and its impact on successful communication: A qualitative analysis* [Poster presentation]. Annual Convention of the American Speech-Language-Hearing Association, Washington, D.C.

Hunter, L., Pring, T., & Martin, S. (1991). The use of strategies to increase speech intelligibility in cerebral palsy: An experimental evaluation. *International Journal of Language and Communication Disorders, 26*(2), 163–174. https://doi.org/10.3109/13682829109012001

Hustad, K. C., Auker, J., Natale, N., & Carlson, R. (2003). Improving intelligibility of speakers with profound dysarthria and cerebral palsy.

Augmentative and Alternative Communication, 19(3), 187–198. https://doi
.org/10.1080/0743461031000121052

Hustad, K. C., & Cahill, M. A. (2003). Effects of presentation mode and repeated familiarization on intelligibility of dysarthric speech. *American Journal of Speech-Language Pathology, 12*(2), 198–208. https://doi.org/10.1044/1058-0360(2003/066)

Hustad, K. C., & Weismer, G. (2007). A continuum of interventions for individuals with dysarthria: Compensatory and rehabilitative treatment approaches. In G. Weismer (Ed.), *Motor speech disorders: Essays for Ray Kent* (pp. 261–303). Plural Publishing.

Johansson, I.-L., Samuelsson, C., & Müller, N. (2020). Patients' and communication partners' experiences of communicative changes in Parkinson's disease. *Disability and Rehabilitation, 42*(13), 1835–1843. https://doi.org/10.1080/09638288.2018.1539875

Johnson, B., Abraham, M., Conway, J., Simmons, L., Edgman-Levitan, S., Sodomka, P., . . . Ford, D. (2008). Partnering with patients and families to design a patient-and family-centered health care system: Recommendations and promising practices. *Institute for Family-Centered Care and the Institute for Healthcare Improvement.* http://www.ihi.org/resources/Pages/Publica
tions/PartneringwithPatientsandFamiliesRecommendationsPromisingPrac
tices.aspx

Jones, W., Mathy, P., Azuma, T., & Liss, J. M. (2004). The effect of aging and synthetic topic cues on the intelligibility of dysarthric speech. *Augmentative and Alternative Communication, 20*(1), 22–29. https://doi.org/10.108
0/07434610310001615981

Kahneman, D. (1973). *Attention and effort.* Prentice-Hall.

Keintz, C. K., Bunton, K., & Hoit, J. D. (2007). Influence of visual information on the intelligibility of dysarthric speech. *American Journal of Speech-Language Pathology, 16*(3), 222–234. https://doi.org/10.1044/1058-0360(2007/027)

Kim, H., & Nanney, S. (2014). Familiarization effects on word intelligibility in dysarthric speech. *Folia Phoniatrica et Logopaedica, 66*(6), 258–264. https://doi.org/10.1159/000369799

Klasner, E. R., & Yorkston, K. M. (2005). Speech intelligibility in ALS and HD dysarthria: The everyday listener's perspective. *Journal of Medical Speech-Language Pathology, 13*(2), 127–139.

Landa, S., Pennington, L., Miller, N., Robson, S., Thompson, V., & Steen, N. (2014). Association between objective measurement of the speech intelligibility of young people with dysarthria and listener ratings of ease of understanding. *International Journal of Speech-Language Pathology, 16*(4), 408–416. https://doi.org/10.3109/17549507.2014.927922

Lansford, K. L., Borrie, S. A., & Barrett, T. S. (2019). Regularity matters: Unpredictable speech degradation inhibits adaptation to dysarthric speech. *Journal of Speech, Language, and Hearing Research, 62*(12), 4282–4290. https://doi.org/10.1044/2019_JSLHR-19-00055

Lansford, K. L., Borrie, S. A., Barrett, T. S., & Flechaus, C. (2020). When additional training isn't enough: Further evidence that unpredictable speech inhibits adaptation. *Journal of Speech, Language, and Hearing Research*, *63*(3), 1700–1711. https://doi.org/10.1044/2020_JSLHR-19-00380

Lansford, K. L., Borrie, S. A., & Bystricky, L. (2016). Use of crowdsourcing to assess the ecological validity of perceptual training paradigms in dysarthria. *American Journal of Speech-Language Pathology*, *25*(2), 233–239. https://doi.org/10.1044/2015_AJSLP-15-0059

Lansford, K. L., Liss, J. M., Caviness, J. N., & Utianski, R. L. (2011). A cognitive–perceptual approach to conceptualizing speech intelligibility deficits and remediation practice in hypokinetic dysarthria. *Parkinson's Disease*, *2011*, Article 150962. https://doi.org/10.4061/2011/150962

Lee, Y., Sung, J. E., & Sim, H. (2014). Effects of listeners' working memory and noise on speech intelligibility in dysarthria. *Clinical Linguistics & Phonetics*, *28*(10), 785–795. https://doi.org/10.3109/02699206.2014.904443

Lemke, U., & Besser, J. (2016) Cognitive load and listening effort: Concepts and age-related considerations. *Ear and Hearing*, *37*(Suppl. 1), 77S–84S. https://doi.org/10.1097/AUD.0000000000000304

Levitan, R., Gravano, A., Wilson, L., Benus, S., Hirschberg, J., & Nenkova, A. (2012). Acoustic-prosodic entrainment and social behavior. In *Proceedings of the North American Chapter of the Association for Computational Linguistics: Human Language Technologies* (pp. 11–19).

Levitan, R., & Hirschberg, J. (2011). Measuring acoustic-prosodic entrainment with respect to multiple levels and dimensions. In *Proceedings of speech* (pp. 3081–3084).

Lindblom B. (1990) Explaining phonetic variation: A sketch of the H&H theory. In W. J. Hardcastle & A. Marchal (Eds.), NATO ASI Series (Series D: Behavioural and Social Sciences). *Speech production and speech modelling* (Vol. 55, pp. 403–439). Springer. https://doi.org/10.1007/978-94-009-2037-8_16

Liss, J. M. (2007). The role of speech perception in motor speech disorders. In G. Weismer (Ed.), *Motor speech disorders: Essays for Ray Kent* (pp. 187–219). Plural Publishing.

Liss, J. M., Spitzer, S. M., Caviness, J. N., & Adler, C. (2002). The effects of familiarization on intelligibility and lexical segmentation in hypokinetic and ataxic dysarthria. *The Journal of Acoustical Society of America*, *112*(6), 3022–3030. https://doi.org/10.1121/1.1515793

Local, J. (2007). Phonetic detail and the organization of talk interaction. In *Proceedings of the 16th International Congress of Phonetic Sciences* (pp. 6–10).

Louwerse, M. M., Dale, R., Bard, E. G., & Jeuniaux, P. (2012). Behavior matching in multimodal communication is synchronized. *Cognitive Science*, *36*(8), 1404–1426. https://doi.org/10.1111/j.1551-6709.2012.01269.x

McAuliffe, M. J., Gibson, E. M., Kerr, S. E., Anderson, T., & LaShell, P. J. (2013). Vocabulary influences older and younger listeners' processing of dysarthric speech. *The Journal of the Acoustical Society of America*, *134*(2), 1358–1368. https://doi.org/10.1121/1.4812764

McCoy, S. L., Tun, P. A., Cox, L. C., Colangelo, M., Stewart, R. A., & Wingfield, A. (2005). Hearing loss and perceptual effort: Downstream effects on older adults' memory for speech. *The Quarterly Journal of Experimental Psychology: Human Experimental Psychology, 58*(1), 22–33. https://doi.org/10.1080/02724980443000151

McFarland, D. H. (2001). Respiratory markers of conversational interaction. *Journal of Speech, Language, and Hearing Research, 44*(1), 128–143. https://doi.org/10.1044/1092-4388(2001/012)

Miller, N. (2013). Measuring up to speech intelligibility. *International Journal of Language & Communication Disorders, 48*(6), 601–612. https://doi.org/10.1111/1460-6984.12061

Miller, N., Allcock, L., Jones, D., Noble, E., Hildreth, A. J., & Burn, D. J. (2007). Prevalence and pattern of perceived intelligibility changes in Parkinson's disease. *Journal of Neurology, Neurosurgery, and Psychiatry, 78*(11), 1188–1190. https://doi.org/10.1136/jnnp.2006.110171

Nagle, K. F., & Eadie, T. L. (2012). Listener effort for highly intelligible tracheoesophageal speech. *Journal of Communication Disorders, 45*(3), 235–245. https://doi.org/10.1016/j.jcomdis.2012.01.001

Nagle, K. F., & Eadie, T. L. (2018). Perceived listener effort as an outcome measure for disordered speech. *Journal of Communication Disorders, 73,* 34–49. https://doi.org/10.1016/j.jcomdis.2018.03.003

Natale, M. (1975). Convergence of mean vocal intensity in dyadic communication as a function of social desirability. *Journal of Personality and Social Psychology, 32*(5), 790–804. https://doi.org/10.1037/0022-3514.32.5.790

Neumann, R., & Stack, F. (2000). "Mood contagion": The automatic transfer of mood between persons. *Journal of Personality and Social Psychology, 79*(2), 211–223. https://doi.org/10.1037/0022-3514.79.2.211

Niederhoffer, K. G., & Pennebaker, J. W. (2002). Linguistic style matching in social interaction. *Journal of Language and Social Psychology, 21*(4), 337–360. https://doi.org/10.1177/026192702237953

Olmstead, A. J., Lee, J., & Viswanathan, N. (2020). The role of the speaker, the listener, and their joint contributions during communicative interactions: A tripartite view of intelligibility in individuals with dysarthria. *Journal of Speech, Language, and Hearing Research, 63*(4), 1106–1114. https://doi.org/10.1044/2020_JSLHR-19-00233

Pardo, J. S. (2006). On phonetic convergence during conversational interaction. *The Journal of the Acoustical Society of America, 119*(4), 2382–2393. https://doi.org/10.1121/1.2178720

Park, J. M. (2012). *Effects of utterance, listener's working memory capacity on speech intelligibility and listening strategies in spastic dysarthria due to cerebral palsy* [Unpublished master's thesis]. Ewha Womans University.

Pickering, M. J., & Garrod, S. (2004). The interactive-alignment model: Developments and refinements. *Behavioral and Brain Sciences, 27*(2), 212–225. https://doi.org/10.1017/S0140525X04450055

Porcaro, C. K., Evitts, P. M., King, N., Hood, C., Campbell, E., White, L., & Veraguas, J. (2020). Effect of dysphonia and cognitive-perceptual listener strategies on speech intelligibility. *Journal of Voice, 34*(5), 806.e7–806.e18. https://doi.org/10.1016/j.jvoice.2019.03.013

Reitter, D., Moore, J. D., & Keller, F. (2006). Priming of syntactic rules in task-oriented dialogue and spontaneous conversation. In R. Sun & N. Miyake (Eds.), In *Proceedings of the 28th Annual Conference of the Cognitive Science Society* (Vol 28, pp. 685–690). Cognitive Science Society.

Richardson, M. J., Marsh, K. L., & Schmit, R. (2005). Effects of visual and verbal interaction on unintentional interpersonal coordination. *Journal of Experimental Psychology: Human Perception and Performance, 31*(1), 62–79. https://doi.org/10.1037/0096-1523.31.1.62

Schegloff, E. A., Jefferson, G., & Sacks, H. (1977). The preference for self-correction in the organization of repair in conversation. *Language, 53*(2), 361–382. https://doi.org/10.2307/413107

Shockley, K., Santana, M. -V., & Fowler, C. A. (2003). Mutual interpersonal postural constraints are involved in cooperative conversation. *Journal of Experimental Psychology: Human Perception and Performance, 29*(2), 326–332. https://doi.org/10.1037/0096-1523.29.2.326

Spitzer, S. M., Liss, J. M., Caviness, J. N., & Adler, C. (2000). An exploration of familiarization effects in the perception of hypokinetic and ataxic dysarthric speech. *Journal of Medical Speech-Language Pathology, 8*(4), 285–293.

Tjaden, K., & Liss, J. M. (1995). The influence of familiarity on judgments of treated speech. *American Journal of Speech-Language Pathology, 4*(1), 39–48. https://doi.org/10.1044/1058-0360.0401.39

Utianski, R. L., Lansford, K. L., Liss, J. M., & Azuma, T. (2011). The effects of topic knowledge on intelligibility and lexical segmentation in hypokinetic and ataxic dysarthria. *Journal of Medical Speech-Language Pathology, 19*(4), 25–36.

Weismer, G., & Martin, R. E. (1992). Acoustic and perceptual approaches to the study of intelligibility. In R. D. Kent (Ed.), *Intelligibility in speech disorders: Theory, measurement and management* (pp. 68–118). John Benjamins.

World Health Organization. (2001). *International Classification of Functioning, Disability, and Health.* https://www.who.int/standards/classifications /international-classification-of-functioning-disability-and-health

Yorkston, K. M., Baylor, C. R., Dietz, J., Dudgeon, B. J., Eadie, T., Miller, R. M., & Amtmann, D. (2008). Developing a scale of communicative participation: A cognitive interviewing study. *Disability and Rehabilitation, 30*(6), 425–433. https://doi.org/10.1080/09638280701625328

Yorkston, K. M., Miller, R. M., & Strand, E. A. (2004). *Management of speech and swallowing disorders in degenerative disease* (2nd ed.). Pro-Ed.

Yorkston, K. M., Strand, E. A., & Kennedy, M. R. (1996). Comprehensibility of dysarthric speech: Implications for assessment and treatment planning. *American Journal of Speech-Language Pathology, 5*(1), 55–66. https://doi .org/10.1044/1058-0360.0501.55

ZOOM Video Communications, Inc. (2020). *ZOOM* (Version 5.0.4) [Computer software]. https://zoom.us/support/download

APPENDIX 7–1

Checklist for Listener Strategies to Maximize Understanding

Checklist for Listener Strategies
☐ Use active listening skills 　☐ Focus on speaker 　☐ Keep on topic 　☐ Use repair strategies when needed
☐ Watch for signs a communication is starting
☐ Observe for signs of topic change
☐ Find out the topic
☐ Use cues from the speaker's face, body, and gestures
☐ Use all modalities to repair breakdowns 　☐ Spoken 　☐ Written 　☐ Gestures 　☐ Alphabet Board
☐ Make sure your ears and eyes are performing optimally
☐ Provide encouragement and feedback to the speaker
☐ Schedule important discussions for ideal conditions ☐ Discuss rules for interaction with the speaker

CHAPTER 8

Strategies to Alter the Communication Environment for Better Understanding

Key Points:

- Variables within the communication environment can either hinder or assist effective communication for speakers with reduced intelligibility.

- Clients and their communication partners should actively identify barriers in their communication environment.

- When using technology, audio settings can be adjusted to allow for maximum signal from the speaker and minimal background noise

- Modifications to the communication environment can be simple to implement and may improve the speaker's intelligibility greatly.

Beyond the behaviors of the speaker and listener, the International Classification of Functioning, Disability, and Health (ICF) reminds us to consider other factors that may influence a communication exchange (World Health Organization, 2001). Environmental factors are "external to the person and can be either a positive or negative influence on the individual's interaction and performance in society" (Threats, 2007, p. 68). The ICF also focuses on personal factors, which can include a person's attitude, experiences, and education. These factors may relate to either speaker or listener. This chapter focuses on environmental, rather than personal factors, but Threats (2007) provides useful insight into both factors related to clients dealing with neurogenic communication disorders.

We consider environmental factors described in the ICF to be facilitators that assist a person's functioning or barriers that limit their functioning (World Health Organization, 2001). Threats (2007) makes the important point that removing barriers does not always facilitate a person's functioning. We need to focus both on removing barriers and finding ways to facilitate communicative success. This chapter covers environmental factors, including the physical and social environment, where our clients are participating in real-life communication situations. This may include various settings such as home, school, workplace, and the client's community. In the ICF model, contextual factors related to the communicative environment may improve intelligibility and comprehensibility.

IDENTIFYING ENVIRONMENTAL BARRIERS

Clinicians should instruct both our clients and their listeners in ways to identify barriers that are present in their communicative environments. Berry and Sanders (1983) suggested that we work with clients to consider amplifiers that assist communication as well. The Situational Intelligibility Survey (SIS) is an evaluation protocol that clients and/or their listeners can use to describe barriers and amplifiers in their environment. This protocol consists of a list of up to 25 different communication situations that are scored according to the level of difficulty of understanding the client's speech. We can customize the protocol to include situations specific to the client, which may assist the SLP in making specific recommendations for improving the communicative environment. You can find the SIS protocol in Appendix 8–1. The Perceptual Dysarthria Evaluation (PDE) protocol contains several questions related to the client's communication in different environmental settings, including visual, auditory, and distance from others (Swigert, 2010). If used over time, the PDE protocol can document how well adjustments help improve listener understanding. Use of telepractice may be an excellent way to determine environmental barriers while your clients remain in their home for sessions.

APPROACHES FOR DEALING WITH COMMUNICATIVE NOISE

In the process of communication, noise is anything that distracts from the signal being understood by the listener. As discussed in Chapter 1, Rothwell (2016) mentions four kinds of noise that could influence a communication exchange, including physiological, psychological, semantic, and physical. Each is discussed here briefly, along with examples related to adult clients, their listeners, and their communicative environment. Physical noise related to the environment and strategies related to reducing barriers and facilitating communication are covered with more depth.

Physiological Noise

Physiological noise occurs when a physical impairment disrupts communication. Chapters 2 and 7 cover challenges related to speech impairment and listener impairment due to hearing loss. We can work with our clients to reduce the impact of physiological noise by improving speech through a subsystem approach (Chapter 5), speaker-specific intelligibility and comprehensibility strategies (Chapter 6), and listener strategies (Chapter 7).

Psychological Noise

Bias or assumptions are forms of psychological noise that can interfere with a message communicated between a speaker and listener. If a listener views a speaker with a communication disorder as less capable or knowledgeable, they are making an assumption that may interfere with communication.

Threats (2007) discusses whether clinicians are barriers or facilitators with our clients. We believe we are facilitating communication, but we may form bias or assumptions regarding the extent of treatment our client needs or how they should feel about their disorder. Many of us have worked with clients who were challenging because they may not have been as motivated as we expected. These feelings can color our communication and treatment planning with clients, where, for optimal success, we want their input.

Semantic Noise

Semantic noise interferes with communication when the speaker and listener do not share a language code or experience. Reduction of semantic noise is likely if speakers use the strategies discussed in Chapter 6.

Providing the listener with context, gestures, or visual cues will allow the listener to bypass any semantic noise that occurs due to the speaker's reduced intelligibility. Further, if the communicative partners have planned how to approach communication breakdowns and repairs (Chapters 6 and 7), the impact of semantic noise will be lessened.

Physical Noise

When something external to either the speaker or listener interferes with the transmission of the message, we refer to this as physical noise. At times, we can alter our environment to reduce the impact or even completely eliminate physical noise. However, there are some types of physical noise we cannot control. We can also adapt to the physical environment to increase our chances of understanding a message. Both speakers and listeners can use adaptations and environmental modifications to improve communication.

ADAPTATION TO ENVIRONMENT

Research has shown us we can adapt to noisy environments to enhance communication. Listeners can use selective listening to attend to one person when there are other voices and noises nearby. The "cocktail party effect" is one example of an adaptation to a noisy environment that has been described for many years in research studies (Arons, 1992; Cherry, 1953). Listeners who are in a noisy situation with competing voices can selectively focus on one speaker's voice above the other noise. Studies on selective listening have found that listeners can focus on one person's speech signal when presented with signals from multiple speakers (Bronkhorst, 2000). Most of us can recall a situation where you had to focus on one speaker in a crowd of people talking and know it takes some effort to do this. If you are interested in what the person is saying, you will focus on that. If not, you may zone out and miss information. We can discuss this ability with our client's communicative partners to help them realize there may be times when they need to focus to hear their partner over other noises.

Speakers also have adaptations to improve communication in noise. When speakers use a louder voice when communicating in noisy conditions, this is called the Lombard effect (Junqua, 1993; Lombard, 1911). Junqua (1993) found that non-disordered speakers achieve this louder condition by increasing loudness, but also by increasing pitch and reducing speech rate. Clear speech, discussed earlier in Chapter 5 applies the Lombard effect in part to assist speakers to increase intelligibility (Skowronski & Harris, 2006).

It is important to remember that the Lombard effect occurs in non-disordered speakers, but these effects are not the same in individuals with speech and voice disorders. Background noise reduces intelligibility of individuals with Parkinson's disease compared to speakers with non-disordered speech (Adams et al., 2008; Chiu & Forrest, 2018; Leszcz, 2012). McAuliffe and colleagues reported that background noise had different impacts on intelligibility across speakers with dysarthria. Additionally, reduced intelligibility in background noise has been noted in alaryngeal speakers using tracheoesophageal speech (TES) (McColl et al., 1998) as well in alaryngeal speakers using esophageal speech (ES), electrolaryngeal speech (EL), and TES (Holley et al., 1983) compared to typical laryngeal speakers. Background noise has reduced intelligibility in speakers with dysphonia compared to non-disordered speakers (Ishikawa et al., 2017). Individuals with dysphonia frequently report reduced intelligibility, particularly in noisy environments (Jacobson et al., 1997; Smith et al., 1998).

The impact of background noise on intelligibility in individuals with Parkinson's disease varies with dysarthria severity (Rountrey, 2020). Results of this study revealed that as noise increased, speakers in the more severe, less intelligible group had improved intelligibility. Speakers who were less severe and more intelligible demonstrated a reduction of intelligibility with background noise. Rountrey and colleagues (2020) speculated that the Lombard effect impacted loudness, pitch, and rate of content words in the lower intelligibility group. They reasoned that the reduced intelligibility in the higher intelligibility group was due to the effects of the background noise on the listener. These results are interesting and we may learn more about how background noise impacts intelligibility over time, but most studies have shown background noise is not helpful to speakers with reduced intelligibility. For the most part, our clients can't rely on the Lombard effect to assist them in being understood by listeners. Given that, SLPs should work with clients and their communicative partners to modify environmental factors to enhance communication.

ENVIRONMENTAL MODIFICATION

Both speakers and listeners can change their behaviors to enhance intelligibility and comprehensibility. Threats (2002) notes that although environmental factors relate to participation in the ICF model (World Health Organization, 2001), there is limited research examining application of focusing on the environment and efficacy of intervention with neurogenic clients. Many of the modification strategies involve application of common sense and increased attention to the communication process. Discussion of ways to modify the environment involving both your client and their listeners is a good start. It may be helpful to have them practice these modifications with SLP feedback.

Improving Proximity Between Speakers and Listeners

Speakers and listeners should make efforts to be close together during conversations. This seems obvious, but we often try to communicate a message to someone in another room, down the hallway, or just across the room. For speakers with reduced intelligibility, having their voice be even quieter due to distance from the listener is a disadvantage. The American National Standards Institute (ANSI) standards (Acoustic Society of America, 1977) for rating speech interference based on noise show that in non-disordered adults, speakers using normal loudness should not be farther than four feet from listeners in an outside environment. Berry and Sanders (1983) suggest that indoor settings may have even more auditory noise and challenges for listeners. They state that we cannot stress the impact of being close to listeners enough. Having only a small distance between communicative partners allows the listener to gain visual information, as well as hearing a louder voice because there is less distance between them. Both listeners and speakers should be trained to make efforts to be in the same room and sit facing each other, when possible.

Reducing or Eliminating Background Noise

Because we know that noise has a detrimental effect on disordered speech, it's important for our speakers and listeners to choose a quiet environment for communication. If you can control a noise, that is useful, but if not, then move away from it. In the home, there are noises we live with every day that can be reduced or eliminated. Turn off television, radios, as well as noisy fans and appliances (Yoho & Borrie, 2018; Duffy, 2019). If there is noise coming in from outside, close doors and windows or move away from them. When clients leave home, they should find the quietest places to communicate when possible. Requesting a table away from the kitchen or areas of high noise level could boost their ability to be heard. If they are attending a concert or movie, they should work out a gesture or signal to let their communicative partner know they need refreshments. If a signal is established in advance, the communication will be more effective because the listener already knows what is needed, or at least knows a verbal message with specific information is coming.

Improving Access to Visual Information

Listeners gain information from a speaker's facial movements during speech (Barkmeier, 1988; Evitts et al., 2009; Evitts et al., 2016; Hunter et al., 1991; Hustad & Cahill, 2003; Keintz et al., 2007), as well as from gestures (Garcia & Cannito, 1996a, 1996b). To make the most of this visual information, listeners must be able to see the speaker well. Sitting close together will be a good start. We can suggest that our speakers avoid being backlit by having bright light behind them which may make it difficult to see them (Clark, 2019). Dim lighting will also add to the challenge, so encourage communicative partners to sit in well-lit environments. Both speaker and listener should have good lighting around their face to allow their partner to take full advantage of visual information related to the message (Berry & Sanders, 1983).

Reducing or Eliminating Distractions

Either communicative partner can become distracted during a conversation. We've discussed eliminating auditory background noise, which would be a major distraction. If either partner is visually focused on something else, such as a phone or computer screen, then that is a distraction that takes away from the speaker's message. Clinicians should coach their clients and communicative partners to avoid multitasking during important conversations to improve understanding.

Using External Aids

External aids can be useful when needed. Listeners who use hearing aids should make sure they are working at all times (Chapter 7). Speakers may need to use amplification for situations where they have to speak over a crowd, such as giving a speech or running a meeting. SLPs can work with clients to make the most of the amplification. Disordered speech that is amplified will just be louder, not more intelligible, which means clients may have to work on other speech parameters before using amplification successfully.

Speaking Clearly When Wearing Face Masks

Now that many people are wearing masks during communication, many of us have no doubt noticed that it seems to be more difficult to understand people who wear masks. Studies investigating the effects of masks on the speaker's signal and intelligibility back up this perception. Masks can impact clear and effective communication due to reduced visual access to speech movements and muffling of speech sounds (Kim & Thompson, 2021). Studies have shown that masks act as acoustic filters and decrease intensity (loudness) of the speaker. Goldin and colleagues (2020) found that intensity decreased by 3 to 4 dB in speakers wearing surgical masks and by 9 to 12 dB in speakers wearing N95 masks. Atcherson and colleagues (2020) examined the impact on intensity for speakers wearing masks only, compared to masks plus a transparent shield. They found that surgical-type masks reduced intelligibility between 5 to 10 dB, and that adding a transparent shield along with the mask to reduce intensity up to 29 dB. In non-disordered speakers, masks were found to reduce intelligibility but use of clear speech strategies by the speakers improved intelligibility (Kim & Thompson, 2021). Many of us can probably relate to feeling less intelligible when wearing a mask in our everyday communication. It is likely that our clients with reduced intelligibility feel this impact much more than we do. Encouraging them to use strategies and management techniques described in Chapters 5 and 6, especially clear speech, is supported by studies on the impact of masks.

Using the Phone Effectively

When we use a telephone to communicate, the speech signal can be degraded by noise from three sources. Skowronski and Harris (2006) describe acoustic noise in the speaker's environment, channel noise which is electronic echo or noises in the phone itself, and acoustic noise in the listener's environment. There's a reason people used to stand in a phone booth to make a call. Our cordless and cell phones are now used in all environments with little thought given to the noise level on the end of either person on the call. SLPs can prepare clients to use their phone in the best possible way to enhance communication. Remind your client that background noise on the phone can be very distracting to their listener (Kleijn et al., 2015). Having both users of the phone talk in a quiet environment is not only polite, but is likely to improve intelligibility during the call.

Adjusting Audio Settings for Video Chat Communication

For clients who are using video chat communication environments like ZOOM, Skype, and FaceTime, we can make adjustments to improve the channel that the signal moves through. Both speaker and listener should adjust to their physical environment to facilitate better sound quality. Many people have learned how to use online communication for meetings and calls to friends and family. SLPs can instruct their clients and their communicative partners to use common sense strategies to improve the channel for auditory signals. Starting with a quiet background environment can be helpful, which can involve turning off TVs, fans, and staying away from noisy family or pets. If they can go into a room and close the door, that is ideal. Joining from a car, restaurant, or outside environment will add background noise that will make it harder for listeners to hear. Having a strong Internet signal will reduce sound and visual distortions. It's also a good idea to mute your own microphone when you are not speaking. For useful information on creating an optimal acoustic remote environment, interested clinicians can review Schneider et al. (2021).

The starting point when using video chat is ensuring that the microphone works well. Both communicative partners should check their audio system using the platform's specifications. If the built-in microphone on the computer is not ideal, headphones with a microphone may provide a better signal. When using ZOOM, there is an option to have the audio signal from a phone call and that may provide the best channel for a speaker's message. There are settings within each type of video conference or video chat that can be changed to enhance the speaker's signal. Both speakers and listeners should be sure to adjust these to ensure the best audio signal (Grillo et al., 2021). Specific instructions will not be provided here, as it is likely websites and terms may evolve over time, but the following sections will contain basic information on what alterations may be possible for video conferencing or chat.

ZOOM Audio Settings

Instructions for ZOOM audio settings can be useful in helping clients improve audio signal for their listeners. Information can be found at the following website: https://support.zoom.us/hc/en-us/articles/360046244692 -Background-noise-suppression?mobile_site=true SLPs can assist their clients to find the audio settings in ZOOM that will allow them to modify settings. Currently, in ZOOM, there are several levels of background noise suppression that can be selected. These levels include:

1. Auto: This is the default setting that provides a moderate level of background noise reduction. This setting automatically adjusts for background noise as it changes. It will not adjust for music in the background.

2. Low: This setting provides minimal noise reduction. Low levels of consistent background noise will be blocked.

3. Medium: This setting is optimal for eliminating background noise in the environment, such as fan noise.

4. High: This is the highest level of noise reduction which will eliminate typing and noise from crumpling papers.

A trial-and-error approach may allow you to work with your client in their home environment to determine which settings are best for their needs.

Based on clinical experience with voice clients, Grillo and colleagues (2021) suggest using the low noise reduction setting, along with checking the box that ensures original sound will be used.

Smart Phone or Tablet Audio Settings

For clients who may use their smart phones or tablets to video chat with family or friends, there are audio adjustments that may enhance the audio signal. Audio settings can be modified in the control center of FaceTime and you can find directions at the following link: https://www.techrepub lic.com/article/ios-15-tip-how-to-reduce-distractions-and-increase-audio -quality-in-facetime/ Two choices for audio in FaceTime include:

1. Wide spectrum audio mode: This setting provides audio that is the most representative of the environment and does not prioritize background or voice.

2. Voice isolation mode: Voice is prioritized over background noise. This setting will mute background noise as much as possible.

Based on the descriptions above, the voice isolation mode may be the best setting for your client who wants to use video chat. Trying both options when the client is in their home environment will help you determine this.

Skype Audio Settings

If your client uses Skype to communicate with others, there are setting modifications that can enhance the audio signal. Settings adjustments for Skype noise cancellation include:

1. Auto: This is the default setting and the Skype app will use the environment to adjust the level of noise.

2. Low: This setting suppresses low levels of consistent background noise, such as from a fan.

3. High: All background noise will be reduced except for speech sounds.

4. Off: No noise cancellation will occur.

The high noise cancellation setting may be the most effective for clients using Skype, but this can be determined by trying the levels out in the client's environment. Information on these levels and adjustments (Bohon, 2021) can be found at https://support.skype.com/en/faq/FA34863/how-do -i-change-audio-and-video-settings-in-skype-on-desktop

IMPACT OF COMMUNICATIVE ENVIRONMENT ON SPEAKERS WITH HEAD AND NECK CANCER

We know that background noise is part of daily life in most communication situations and that it can reduce intelligibility, even in non-disordered speakers. Due to reduced loudness, altered voice quality, and other factors, background noise has a negative impact on the intelligibility of alaryngeal speakers, regardless of the type of communication they use (Eadie et al., 2016). Challenging communication environments for individuals with H&N cancer include using the phone, speaking over noise, in the car, or outdoors (Childes et al., 2017). Eadie and colleagues (2016) remind us that those individuals with H&N cancer may only have mild speech impairments, such as sound distortions, but will find that even low levels of background noise can be detrimental to intelligibility. McColl and colleagues (1998) found that both TEP speakers and non-disordered speakers had lower intelligibility scores when background noise was introduced, but intelligibility was more reduced by the noise in the TEP speakers than the healthy speakers. Similar findings of reduced intelligibility in noise have been documented in EL speakers as well (Cox et al., 2020; Holley et al., 1983).

Doyle and Keith (2005) remind us that alaryngeal speakers may become fairly intelligible in their typical settings with familiar listeners, but in real-world situations, they will interact with unfamiliar listeners, often in the presence of background noise. Speakers who have been treated for H&N cancer will benefit from practicing all the environmental modifications previously described in this chapter. Doyle and Finchem (2019) state that reminding communicative partners that alaryngeal speech, specifically ES, has a reduced loudness level, which allows more impact of background noise. These clients may need to consider the use of devices that may be helpful in certain challenging situations. For example, Childes and colleagues (2017) reported that when clients treated for H&N cancer described environments where their alaryngeal speech was not well understood. These individuals reported that when background noise was present and/or on the phone, they relied on assistance from speech-generating devices (SGD) or teletypewriter devices (TTY). SLPs can discuss these options for clients to improve their communication effectiveness for everyday situations. Addressing strategies to enhance the environment for optimal communication will be a critical step in the management of these individuals.

SUMMARY

The communicative environment can present many challenges for speakers with reduced intelligibility and their listeners. SLPs can work with speakers and listeners to assist them in identifying barriers to communication and amplifiers. Once identified, SLPs can teach both communicative partners to reduce the impact of environmental challenges to understanding. These modifications can include actions the communicative partners can both take, such as sitting closer together and having eye contact. Some modifications might involve reducing distractions or background noise, when possible. Discussing each client's personal circumstances will allow clinicians to assist them in using phones or video chat to help optimize the environment and settings to improve intelligibility. A checklist of environmental modifications is provided in Appendix 8–2. Many of the modifications are quite easy to implement, but our clients will benefit from our assistance with identifying what will help, and practice changing the environment in the best possible way.

 # Case Study

Dysarthria Case: Because Jack had several main environments where communication is critical, including home and college, Christy sat down with him to discuss difficulties he may have in these different settings. She used the Situational Intelligibility Survey (SIS; Berry & Sanders, 1983) to record Jack's reaction to various environments. She discussed the best ways to change the communication environments with Jack and his listeners through remote and in-person meetings. At home, Jack's dad discussed his own hearing loss and how he needed to remember to use his hearing aid. Jack's family mentioned they often speak loudly from different rooms, rather than coming into the room to speak. They all agreed to work on that, along with reducing background noises such as, noise from appliances, and their barking dog. Jack's friends agreed that they often play loud music or have their video games turned up loud and decided muting or turning volume down would help Jack be understood. Jack's instructors decided that classroom environments were difficult for him at times due to background noise from other students talking, chairs moving, and so forth. They all agreed to make a commitment to reduce the noise in their classrooms as much as possible. His instructors felt it was important for Jack to make the effort to come close to them to speak in the classroom. Jack worked with Christy to adjust the settings on his ZOOM (ZOOM Video Communications, Inc., 2020) and FaceTime to maximize his voice over background noises. They also discussed finding a quiet place to make phone calls.

 # Case Study

Voice Disorders Case: Near the end of her course of treatment, Thomas invited Beth's husband and daughter to the session to discuss how all three of them could do their best to improve the environment around their communication with Beth. They discussed making sure they were in the same room with her, rather than yelling down the stairs or into another room to share a message. They all agreed to sit away from the noisy music when they have their weekly pizza dinner out with the grandchildren. One issue they identified was that Beth's young grandchildren often talk loudly over her when she is speaking, to ask questions or comment on the books she reads them. They devised a plan to teach the grandchildren that when "Grammy" is talking, they need to be silent. They will all practice cueing the grandchildren on this. Beth is grateful that her family has actively been involved in helping her improve her voice and the environment where she will be speaking. Thomas feels that because they were involved with identifying possible problems and solutions, it is likely they will follow through to help her in this way.

REFERENCES

Acoustical Society of America. (1977). American national standard for rating noise with respect to speech interference. *American Institute of Physics*, 1–4.

Adams, S., Dykstra, A. D., Jenkins, M. E., & Jog, M. S. (2008). Speech-to-noise levels and conversational intelligibility in hypophonia and Parkinson's disease. *Journal of Medical Speech-language Pathology*, *16*(4), 165–172.

Arons, B. (1992). A review of the cocktail party effect. *Journal of the American Voice I/O Society*, *12*(7), 35–50.

Atcherson, S. R., Finley, E. T., McDowell, B. R., & Watson, C. (2020). More speech degradations and considerations in the search for transparent face coverings during the COVID-19 pandemic. Online feature. *Audiology Today.* July/August 2020.

Barkmeier, J. M. (1988). *Intelligibility of dysarthric speakers: Audio-only and audio-visual presentations.* [Master's thesis, University of Iowa]. Iowa Research Online. https://doi.org/10.17077/etd.dvdycbts

Berry, W. R., & Sanders, S. B. (1983). Environmental education: The universal management approach for adults with dysarthria. In W. R. Berry (Ed.), *Clinical dysarthria* (pp. 202–216). College-Hill Press.

Bohon, C. (2021, August 27). *iOS 15 tip: How to reduce distractions and increase audio quality in FaceTime.* TechRepublic. https://www.techrepublic.com/article/ios-15-tip-how-to-reduce-distractions-and-increase-audio-quality-in-facetime/

Bronkhorst, A. W. (2000). The cocktail party phenomenon: A review of research on speech intelligibility in multiple-talker conditions. *Acta Acustica United with Acustica*, *86*(1), 117–128.

Cherry, E. C. (1953). Some experiments on the recognition of speech, with one and with two ears. *The Journal of the Acoustical Society of America*, *25*(5), 975–979. https://doi.org/10.1121/1.1907229

Childes, J. M., Palmer, A. D., Fried-Oken, M., & Graville, D. J. (2017). The use of technology for phone and face-to-face communication after total laryngectomy. *American Journal of Speech-Language Pathology*, *26*(1), 99–112. https://doi.org/10.1044/2016_AJSLP-14-0106

Chiu, Y.-F., & Forrest, K. (2018). The impact of lexical characteristics and noise on intelligibility on Parkinsonian speech. *Journal of Speech, Language, and Hearing Research*, *61*(4), 837–846. https://doi.org/10.1044/2017_JSLHR-S-17-0205

Clark, H. (2019, April 10). *Treatment of dysarthria in adults with acute, chronic, and degenerative conditions* [PowerPoint slides]. North Carolina Speech-Language and Hearing Association.

Cox, S. R., McNicholl, K., Shadle, C. H., & Chen, W. (2020). Variability of electrolaryngeal speech intelligibility in multitalker babble. *American Journal* of *Speech-Language Pathology, 29*(4), 2012–2022. https://doi.org/10.1044/2020_AJSLP-20-00092

Doyle, P. C., & Finchem, E. (2019). Teaching esophageal speech: A process of collaborative instruction. In P. C. Doyle (Ed.), *Clinical care and rehabilitation in head and neck cancer* (pp. 145–161). Springer. https://doi.org/10.1007/978-3-030-04702-3_10

Doyle, P. C., & Keith, R. L. (Eds.). (2005). *Contemporary consideration in the treatment and rehabilitation of head and neck cancer: Voice, speech, and swallowing.* Pro-Ed.

Duffy, J. R. (2019). *Motor speech disorders: Substrates, differential diagnosis, and management* (4th ed.). Elsevier.

Eadie, T. L., Otero, D. S., Bolt, S., Kapsner-Smith, M., & Sullivan, J. R. (2016). The effect of noise on relationships between speech intelligibility and self-reported communication measures in tracheoesophageal speakers. *American Journal of Speech-Language Pathology, 25*(3), 393–407. https://doi.org/10.1044/2016_AJSLP-15-0081

Evitts, P. M., Starmer, H., Teets, K., Montgomery, C., Calhoun, L., Schulze, A., MacKenzie, J., . . . Adams, L. (2016). The impact of dysphonic voices on healthy listeners: Listener reaction times, speech intelligibility, and listener comprehension. *American Journal of Speech-Language Pathology, 25*(4), 561–575. https://doi.org/10.1044/2016_AJSLP-14-0183

Evitts, P. M., Van Dine, A., & Holler, A. (2009). Effects of audio-visual information and mode of speech on listener perceptions of alaryngeal speakers. *International Journal of Speech-Language Pathology, 11*(6), 450–460. https://doi.org/10.3109/17549500903003078

Garcia, J. M., & Cannito, M. P. (1996a). Influence of verbal and nonverbal context on sentence intelligibility of a speaker with dysarthria. *Journal of Speech, Language, and Hearing Research, 39*(4), 750–760. https://doi.org/10.1044/jshr.3904.750

Garcia, J. M., & Cannito, M. P. (1996b). Top down influences on the intelligibility of a dysarthric speaker: Addition of natural gestures and situational context. In D. A. Robin, K. M. Yorkston, & D. R. Beukelman (Eds.), *Disorders of motor speech* (pp. 89–104). Brookes.

Goldin, A., Weinstein, B. E., & Shiman, N. (2020). How do medical masks degrade speech perception? *Hearing Review, 27*(5), 8–9.

Grillo, E., Petty, B. E., & Zacharias, S. (2021, November 18–20). *Teleprac-tice and technology in voice* [Technical session]. Annual Convention of the American Speech-Language-Hearing Association, Washington D.C.

Holley, S. C., Lerman, J., & Randolph, K. (1983). A comparison of the intelligibility of esophageal, electrolaryngeal, and normal speech in quiet and in noise. *Journal of Communication Disorders, 16*(2), 143–155. https://doi.org/10.1016/0021-9924(83)90045-X

How do I change audio and video settings in Skype on desktop? (n.d.). Skype. https://support.skype.com/en/faq/FA34863/how-do-i-change-audio-and-video-settings-in-skype-on-desktop

Hunter, L., Pring, T., & Martin, S. (1991). The use of strategies to increase speech intelligibility in cerebral palsy: An experimental evaluation. *International Journal of Language & Communication Disorders, 26*(2), 163–174. https://doi.org/10.3109/13682829109012001

Hustad, K. C., & Cahill, M. A. (2003). Effects of presentation mode and repeated familiarization on intelligibility of dysarthric speech. *American Journal of Speech-Language Pathology, 12*(2), 198–208. https://doi.org/10.1044/1058-0360(2003/066)

Ishikawa, K., Boyce, S., Kelchner, L., Powell, M. G., Schieve, H., de Alarcon, A., & Khosla, S. (2017). The effect of background noise on intelligibility of dysphonic speech. *Journal of Speech, Language, and Hearing Research, 60*(7), 1919–1929. https://doi.org/10.1044/2017_JSLHR-S-16-0012

Jacobson, B. H., Johnson, A., Grywalski, C., Silbergleit, A., Jacobson, G., Benninger, M. S., & Newman, C. W. (1997). The Voice Handicap Index (VHI): Development and validation. *American Journal of Speech-Language Pathology, 6*(3), 66–70. https://doi.org/10.1044/1058-0360.0603.66

Junqua, J. -C. (1993). The Lombard reflex and its role on human listeners and automatic speech recognizers. *The Journal of the Acoustical Society of America, 93*(1), 510–524. https://doi.org/10.1121/1.405631

Keintz, C. K., Bunton, K., & Hoit, J. D. (2007). Influence of visual information on the intelligibility of dysarthric speech. *American Journal of Speech-Language Pathology, 16*(3), 222–234. https://doi.org/10.1044/1058-0360(2007/027)

Kim, Y., & Thompson, A. (2021, November 18–20). *Effects of face masks on speech acoustics and intelligibility* [Technical session]. Annual Convention of the American Speech-Language-Hearing Association, Washington D.C.

Kleijn, W. B., Crespo, J. B., Hendriks, R. C., Petkov, P., Sauert, B., & Vary, P. (2015). Optimizing speech intelligibility in a noisy environment. *IEEE Signal Processing Magazine, 32*(2), 43–54. http://doi.org/10.1109/MSP.2014.2365594

Leszcz, T. M. (2012). *The effect of multitalker background noise on speech intelligibility in Parkinson's disease and controls* [Master's thesis, University of Western Ontario]. Electronic Thesis and Dissertation Repository. https://ir.lib.uwo.ca/etd/628

Lombard, E. (1911). Le signe de l'élévation de la voix. *Annales des Maladies de L'Oreille et du Larynx, 37*, 101–119.

McAuliffe, M. J., Schaefer, M., O'Beirne, G. A., & LaPointe, L. L. (2009, November). *Effect of noise upon the perception of speech intelligibility in dysarthria* [Poster presentation]. Annual Convention of the American Speech-Language-Hearing Association, New Orleans, LA.

McColl, D., Fucci, D., Petrosino, L., Martin, D. E., & McCaffrey, P. (1998). Listener ratings of the intelligibility of tracheoesophageal speech in noise. *Journal of Communication Disorders, 31*(4), 279–289. https://doi.org/10.1016/S0021-9924(98)00008-2

Rothwell, J. D. (2016). *In the company of others: An introduction to communication.* (5th ed.). Oxford University Press.

Rountrey, C. E., Yaeger, A., & Coleman, M. (2020). *An examination of the effect of background noise on speech intelligibility in spontaneous Parkinsonian speech* [Research presentation]. Madonna International Motor Speech Disorders Conference, Santa Barbara, CA.

Schneider, S. L., Habich, L., Weston, Z. M., & Rosen, C. A. (2021). Observations and considerations for implementing remote acoustic voice recording and analysis in clinical practice. *Journal of Voice* [Advance online publication]. https://doi.org/10.1016/j.jvoice.2021.06.011

Skowronski, M. D., & Harris, J. G. (2006). Applied principles of clear and Lombard speech for automated intelligibility enhancement in noisy environments. *Speech Communication, 48*(5), 549–558. https://doi.org/10.1016/j.specom.2005.09.003

Smith, E., Taylor, M., Mendoza, M., Barkmeier, J., Lemke, J., & Hoffman, H. (1998). Spasmodic dysphonia and vocal fold paralysis: Outcomes of voice problems on work-related functioning. *Journal of Voice, 12*(2), 223–232. https://doi.org/10.1016/S0892-1997(98)80042-8

Swigert, N. B. (2010). *The source for dysarthria* (2nd ed.). Pro-Ed.

Threats, T. (2002). Evidence-based practice research using the WHO framework. *Journal of Medical Speech-Language Pathology, 10*(3), xvii–xxiv.

Threats, T. (2007). Access for persons with neurogenic communication disorders: Influences of personal and environmental factors of the ICF. *Aphasiology, 21*(1), 67–80. https://doi.org/10.1080/02687030600798303

World Health Organization. (2001). *International Classification of Functioning, Disability, and Health.* https://www.who.int/standards/classifications/international-classification-of-functioning-disability-and-health

Yoho, S. E., & Borrie, S. A. (2018). Combining degradations: The effect of background noise on intelligibility of disordered speech. *The Journal of the Acoustical Society of America, 143*(1), 281–286. https://doi.org/10.1121/1.5021254

ZOOM Video Communications, Inc. (2021, November 1). *Suppressing background noise for videos.* https://support.zoom.us/hc/en-us/articles/360046244692-Background-noise-suppression?mobile_site=true

APPENDIX 8–1

Situational Intelligibility Survey

People have trouble understanding me, him/her: <u>Score</u>

1   Everywhere   _____

2   In noisy places   _____

3   In dark places   _____

4   When strangers are listeners   _____

5   In group conversations   _____

6   When watching TV/listening to radio   _____

7. In stores   _____

8. In restaurants/night spots   _____

9. On the phone   _____

10. While in a car   _____

11. When I am sitting   _____

12. When I am walking   _____

13. When I am tired   _____

14. When I am emotional   _____

15. In the morning   _____

16. In the afternoon   _____

17. At night   _____

18. At a distance of 5 ft (when quiet)   _____

19. At a distance of 10 ft (when quiet)   _____

20. At a distance of 15 ft (when quiet) _____

21. _____ _____

22. _____ _____

23. _____ _____

24. _____ _____

25. _____ _____

Scoring Scale:	All the time	Occasionally	Never
	0	1	2

Total Score = _____

Total Possible = _____

% Score = _____%

Source: Berry and Sanders (1983).

APPENDIX 8–2

Checklist to Maximize Communication Potential by Modifying the Environment

Communication Environment Checklist	
Ensure good proximity between communication partners.	☐ No more than 4 feet outside ☐ Less than 4 feet inside ☐ Adjust as needed for background noise
Reduce background noise by adjusting auditory distractions.	☐ TV ☐ Radio ☐ Fans ☐ Open windows ☐ Talking ☐ Restaurant noise
Improve access to visual information.	☐ Face-to-face positioning ☐ Eye contact ☐ Adequate lighting
Reduce distractions.	☐ Avoid multitasking. ☐ Limit phone or screen access.
Utilize external aids.	☐ Hearing aids for listener ☐ Speech amplification for speaker
Enhance settings.	☐ Phone settings ☐ Video chat settings

Index

Note: Page numbers in **bold** reference non-text material.